Step by Step Manual of Laparoscopic Surgery

LAPAROSCOPIC HERNIA SURGERY

***System requirements*:** 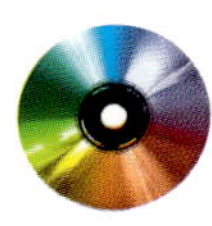

- **Operating System—Windows Vista or above**
- **Web Browser—Google Chrome, Mozilla Firefox, Internet Explorer 9 and above**
- **Essential plugins—Java & Flash player**
    - Facing problems in viewing content—it may be your system does not have Java enabled.
    - If Videos do not show up—it may be the system requires Flash player or need to manage Flash setting. To learn more about Flash setting click on the link in the help section.
    - You can test Java and Flash by using the links from the help section of the CD/DVD.

***Accompanying CD/DVD Rom is playable only in Computer and not in DVD player*.**

CD/DVD has Autorun function—it may take few seconds to load on your computer. If it does not works for you then follow the steps below to access the contents manually:

- Click on My Computer
- Select the CD/DVD drive and click open/explore—this will show list of files in the CD/DVD
- Find and double click file—"launch.html"

For more information about troubleshoot of Autorun click on: http://support.microsoft.com/kb/330135.

Step by Step Manual of Laparoscopic Surgery

LAPAROSCOPIC HERNIA SURGERY

Vol. 4

Series Editors

JS Rajkumar MS FICS Dip. NB (Surg) FRCS (Eng) FRCS (Edin) FRCS (Glasgow) FRCS (Ireland) FIMSA FAIS FRSM (London) FAGE (Gastro) FACG (USA) FICA (USA) FIAGES Dip. MIS (France) AMMC FMAS
Director
Lifeline Institute of Minimal Access Surgery
Advanced lap, Bariatric and Onco-lap Surgeon
No. 47/3 New Avadi Road, Kilpauk
Chennai, Tamil Nadu, India

Neha Shah MS FIAGES FMAS FMIS FAIS FALS
Senior Consultant
Department of GI and Bariatric Surgery
Apollo Nova Specialty Hospitals
Chennai, Tamil Nadu, India

Foreword

CMK Reddy

JAYPEE The Health Sciences Publisher
New Delhi | London | Philadelphia | Panama

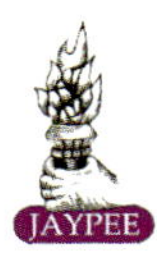

Jaypee Brothers Medical Publishers (P) Ltd

Headquarters

Jaypee Brothers Medical Publishers (P) Ltd
4838/24, Ansari Road, Daryaganj
New Delhi 110 002, India
Phone: +91-11-43574357
Fax: +91-11-43574314
Email: jaypee@jaypeebrothers.com

Overseas Offices

J.P. Medical Ltd
83, Victoria Street, London
SW1H 0HW (UK)
Phone: +44-2031708910
Fax: +02-03-0086180
Email: info@jpmedpub.com

Jaypee-Highlights.
Medical Publishers Inc
City of Knowledge, Bld. 237
Clayton, Panama City, Panama
Phone: +1 507-301-0496
Fax: +1 507-301-0499
Email: cservice@jphmedical.com

Jaypee Medical Inc.
The Bourse
111 South Independence Mall East
Suite 835, Philadelphia
PA 19106, USA
Phone: +1 267-519-9789
Email: jpmed.us@gmail.com

Jaypee Brothers
Medical Publishers (P) Ltd
17/1-B Babar Road, Block-B
Shaymali, Mohammadpur
Dhaka-1207, Bangladesh
Mobile: +08801912003485
Email: jaypeedhaka@gmail.com

Jaypee Brothers
Medical Publishers (P) Ltd
Shorakhute, Kathmandu
Nepal
Phone: +00977-9841528578
Email: jaypee.nepal@gmail.com

Website: www.jaypeebrothers.com
Website: www.jaypeedigital.com

Inquiries for bulk sales may be solicited at: jaypee@jaypeebrothers.com

Step by Step Manual of Laparoscopic Surgery: Laparoscopic Hernia Surgery (Vol. 4)

First Edition: 2016

ISBN 978-93-5152-892-0

Printed at: Ajanta Offset & Packagings Ltd., New Delh

Dedication

We would like to dedicate this series of volumes to our parents, who breathed life into us, nurtured our spirits with confidence and most importantly, taught us values to live by.

Foreword

With rapid advances taking place in every branch of medicine, writing an updated book on any subject is no easy job. With the highly academic background and profound skill in advanced laparoscopic surgery, Prof JS Rajkumar and Dr Neha Shah have ventured to produce step-by-step manuals for various laparoscopic procedures, as excellent reference books for the young endoscopic surgeons as well as those already in practice in the area of minimally invasive surgery.

The first volume of their work is about laparoscopic hernia repair. Each inguinal hernia is so different, our teachers used to say, if one could do a hernia operation confidently, he could do any operation safely. Though open surgery for inguinal hernia is relatively simple, laparoscopic surgery requires lot of experience and reorientation of inguinal anatomy from inside, much more so for recurrent or complicated ones. During the long learning curve, mistakes can occur from the hands of beginners and those working in low volume centres, this book explains those in clear detail, with adequate illustrations, with a primary aim of preventing surgical errors. It is also very important to assimilate the technological advances in laparoscopic instruments, energy sources, meshes and suture material, so that they could find application in appropriate places and situations, for optimal outcome.

It is always difficult to decide how much to say in a situation, while writing a foreword, but with the vast experience of the authors as surgeons and teachers, I am impressed that they could filter the actual required information just appropriate for a junior surgeon. I congratulate the authors for the effort they put in to make this a practical reference book in various common as well as advanced laparoscopic procedures in surgical practice.

Prof CMK Reddy DSc (Hon) FRCS (Glas) FRCS (Ire)
Emeritus Professor of Surgery, TN Dr MGR Medical University
Former Hon Professor of Surgery, Stanley Medical College
President, TN Medical Practitioners' Association and
Indian Chapter, Royal College of Surgeons in Ireland
Examiner to MBBS, MS, MCh (Vasc)
National Board, FRCS and MRCS
Recipient of Dr BC Roy National Award as
Eminent Medical Teacher, General and Vascular Surgeon
Chennai, Tamil Nadu, India

Preface

This series of operative laparoscopy books has been modeled on the immortal Rob and Smith operative surgery line diagram volumes for open surgery. Although there are huge tonnes of laparoscopic surgical books there has been no equivalent to the above mentioned book in minimal invasive surgery. Having operated through laparoscopy for the past 20 years, and being involved in teaching for at least 15 years, we felt that we could attempt to bridge the gap between the theory and the art of minimal access surgery.

Toward this end we felt that a book containing line diagrams and detailing the minutiae of the surgical procedures would help the novice laparoscopist choose his surgical steps with studied confidence. This series is essentially one that provides the complete bandwidth of procedures, starting from diagnostic laparoscopy and going all the way to laparoscopic oncology and bariatric surgery.

In order to enable the reader to understand the steps dynamically, we have also attached a CD/DVD with each volume, in which all the steps of the described operations are shown with a voice over. It is our recommendation that each procedure is seen immediately after the text is perused.

We have divided the subject matter into 14 volumes, that will hopefully cover almost all the available operative surgery spectrum of laparoscopy. You are holding one such volume in your hand.

A final word of advice to our dear readers, you need not buy all the volumes at one go. We would like you to progress in 2 or 3 areas at one time depending on your chosen field of advancement. If you are doing gallbladders already, perhaps you could advance to antireflux surgery or hernioplasty, rather than a single incision colectomy! As you gain experience and exposure you can purchase the next few volumes.

We wish you all the enjoyment and excitement that we have experienced in our learning curves and we hope your curve is much shorter than ours!!!

JS Rajkumar
Neha Shah

Acknowledgments

We would like to thank the following people who have contributed significantly towards making of this book.

Dr Chitrakala Rajkumar, Dr Dilip Chandar, Dr Poornima, Dr Nataraja Sethupathy, Dr Anirudh Rajkumar, Sarvanan, Menaka, Shalini, Meena Kesan, and Akila for helping with the typing of the manuscript.

We thank every single patient who enriched our surgical experience and made us what we are today. And last but not least, we pay our humble respects to the doyens of surgery—the giants upon whose shoulders we dwarves stood and looked at the world. Prof S Vittal, Prof CMK Reddy, and Prof MG Muthukumaraswamy, to mention a few in a golden list.

We would also like to thank Mr Jitendar P Vij (Group Chairman), Mr Ankit Vij (Group President), Ms Chetna Malhotra Vohra (Associate Director), Mr Umar Rashid (Development Editor) and Production team of Jaypee Brothers Medical Publishers (P) Ltd., New Delhi, India.

Contents

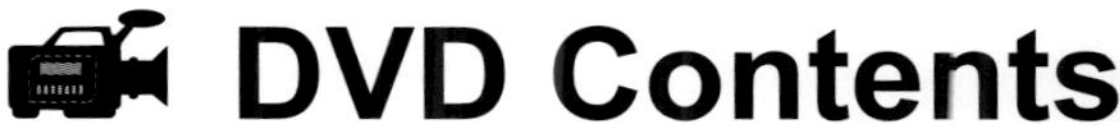

DVD Contents

Chapter 2 video: Laparoscopic TEP

Chapter 3 video: Laparoscopic TAPP

Chapter 5 video: Laparoscopic Para umbilical hernia

Chapter 6 video: Laparoscopic Incisional hernia

Chapter 1

Endoscopic Anatomy of Inguinal Region

INTRODUCTION

It is very important to clearly understand the surgical anatomy of the inguinal region for a safe and successful outcome of laparoscopic hernia repairs.

The laparoscopic view of the groin anatomy is very different from the open one. In laparoscopic hernia repair, we go through a posterior approach while we are used to the anterior approach in open hernia repairs. Changing to a laparoscopic approach requires proper knowledge of anatomy. Certain structures like ilioinguinal nerve, inguinal ligament, pubic tubercle and lacunar ligament are clearly visible in open approach and not so in laparoscopy. Conversely, structures like Cooper's ligament and iliopubic tract that are not visible in the open approach are clearly visible with the laparoscopic approach.

In laparoscopic repair, we are targeting the point of origin of the hernia and not the point of presentation. So laparoscopy deals with all the potential sites at risk for hernia in the groin, i.e. it takes care of direct, indirect, femoral and obturator hernias. However, this is a three-dimensional view with a two-dimensional handycam.

Importance of the Kessler's triangle: The Kessler's triangle is the one between the inguinal ligament and the upper edge of the intersections of the internal oblique, the transversus abdominis muscle and its upper aponeurosis to the rectus sheath. Thus the triangle is medially bounded by the lateral border of the rectus sheath, inferiorly bounded by the inguinal ligament and laterally bounded by the internal oblique transverse section. It is said that when there is a larger Kessler's triangle due to higher intersections of internal oblique and transverses the muscle into the rectus sheath, there is a larger space available for the muscles to occlude the triangle when they contract. This incomplete occlusion is set to be an important anatomical factor in the etiology of inguinal hernia. This triangle is not to be confused with Hasselbach's triangle (*see* below).

HESSELBACH'S TRIANGLE

Frank Hesselbach and Kasper gave an original description of inguinal triangle called Hesselbach's triangle (Fig. 1.1).

Following are the boundaries:

- Superolateral boundary—inferior epigastric vessels
- Medially—rectus sheath (lower third)
- Inferiorly—inguinal ligament (medial third)

MYOPECTINEAL ORIFICE OF FRUCHAUD

In 1956, Henry Fruchaud postulated that all groin hernias essentially originate in a single weak area, which he called the myopectineal orifice. This is funnel-like, and potential space formed superiorly by the internal oblique and transversus abdominis, inferiorly by the superior pubic ramus, medially by the rectus muscle sheath and laterally by the iliopsoas. This entire myopectineal orifice is divided by the iliopubic tract and the inguinal ligament into an inguinal defect (superiorly) and a femoral defect (inferiorly).

This oval, funnel-like potential orifice is formed of the following structures:

- *Superiorly*: Internal oblique and transversus abdominis muscles
- *Inferiorly*: Pecten pubis
- *Medially*: Rectus muscle sheath
- *Laterally*: Iliopsoas muscle

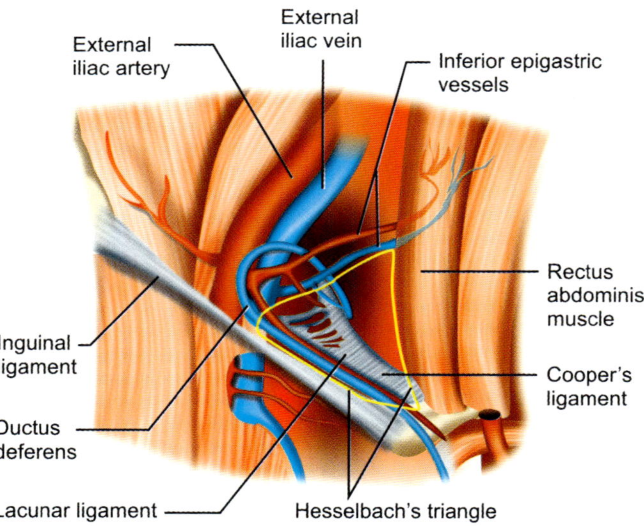

Fig. 1.1: Hesselbach's triangle.

Proper exposure of this orifice is essential to do a proper inguinal hernia repair. The whole orifice is divided by the iliopubic tract into superior and inferior compartments, with the inferior epigastric artery bisecting the superior compartment. Thus, direct and indirect hernias are visualized in the superior compartment and femoral hernias in the inferior compartment (Fig. 1.2).

The superomedial compartment of the myopectineal orifice corresponds to the original Hesselbach's triangle. Covering the complete myopectineal orifice is the anatomical fundamental of laparoscopic hernioplasty.

From the large posterior myopectineal orifice, the inguinal canal funnels forward into a narrow anterior wall, explaining the need for a larger mesh for posterior cover and a much smaller mesh for anterior cover. (15 × 12 cm in laparoscopic repair as it is posterior repair against 6 × 10 cm in open repair of hernia as it is anterior repair).

Peritoneal Landmarks from the Inside

Median Umbilical Ligament

This ligament is present in the midline and runs from the bladder to umbilicus. It represents the obliterated allantoic duct, and the lower part is the site of the rare urachal cyst.

Medial Umbilical Ligament

This ligament represents obliterated umbilical artery on each side and can be traced down to the internal iliac artery.

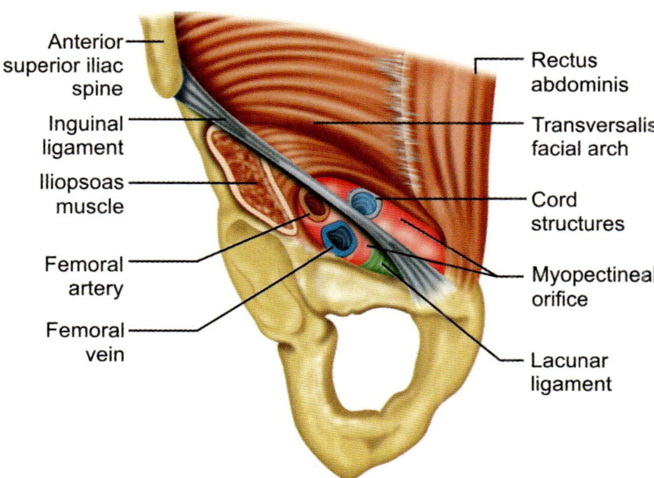

Fig. 1.2: External view of myopectineal orifice of Fruchaud.

Lateral Umbilical Ligament

It is a peritoneal fold which is raised by the inferior epigastric artery and its two veins, and it courses around medial border of internal inguinal ring and passes upwards into the posterior abdominal wall.

FOSSAE

As far as the fossae are concerned, there are three of them that every laparoscopic hernia surgeon should know (Fig. 1.3).

Supravesical Fossa

The infraumbilical area between the median and medial umbilical ligaments is called supravesical fossa. This is the site of origin of the supravesical hernia.

Medial Umbilical Fossa

The infraumbilical area between the medial and lateral umbilical ligaments is called medial umbilical fossae. This is the site of origin of direct inguinal hernias above the iliopubic tract and femoral hernia below the iliopubic tract.

Lateral Umbilical Fossa

The infraumbilical area lateral to the lateral umbilical ligament. This is the site for the origin of the indirect inguinal hernia.

PREPERITONEAL SPACE (FIG. 1.4)

This is a very important space to understand as all the repairs and mesh placement are done in this space.

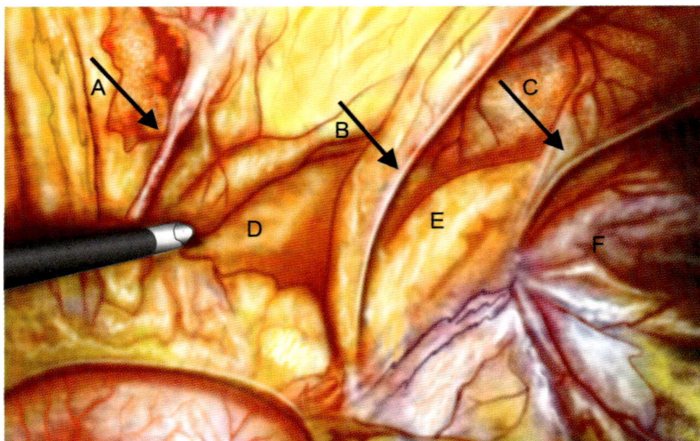

Fig. 1.3: Laparoscopic view of normal pelvic anatomy on the right side (before peritoneal reflection).

Keys: A, median umbilical ligament; B, medial umbilical ligament; C, lateral umbilical ligament; D, supravesical fossa; E, medial fossa; F, lateral fossa.

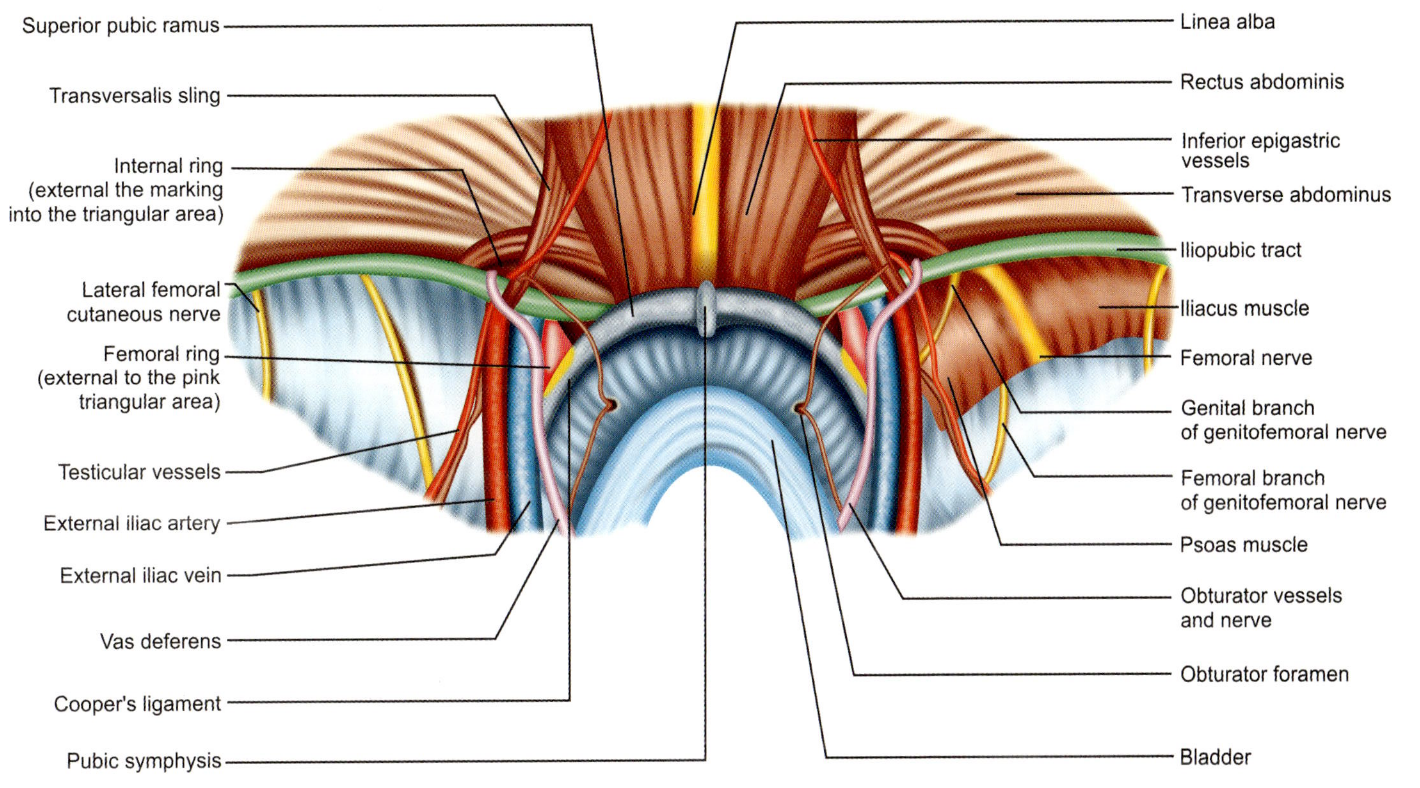

Fig. 1.4: Preperitoneal space.

Bilaminar Transversalis Fascia (of Gallaudet)

The current understanding of the transversalis fascia is of a two layered or bilaminar structure. The superficial layer is a membranous layer and the deep layer is a fatty layer. The superficial layer is closely opposed to the posterior aspect of the rectus abdominis muscle in the posterior rectus sheath. The posterior fatty layer is closely adherent to the underlying peritoneum.

The orientation of the two layers of the transversalis fascia is identical to the two layers of the superficial facia of the anterior abdominal wall as if Camper's and Scarpa's fasciae are reflected inwards.

Both layers are inserted into the Cooper's ligament inferiorly. Condensation of the transversalis fascia forms three important structures: (1) interfoveolar ligament, (2) medial margin of internal ring and (3) iliopubic tract.

Iliopubic Tract (Fig. 1.5)

It is the thickened lateral extension of the transversalis fascia which runs from the superior pubic ramus to the iliopectineal arch and the anterior superior iliac spine.

It forms a strong aponeurotic band only in 28–30% of patients. Its significance in laparoscopic hernia repair is to identify it as it forms the superior border of triangle of pain. No diathermy or tackers are to be used in this triangle.

This continues anteriorly with the forepart of the inguinal ligament, but the tract is distinct in structure and separate from the inguinal ligament. It is anterior to the Cooper's ligament and inferior epigastric artery, and posterior to the inguinal ligament. This separates the internal ring from the

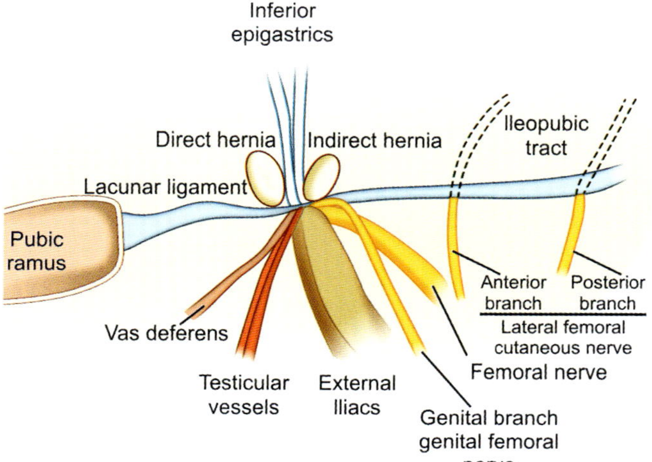

Fig. 1.5: Iliopubic tract.

femoral canal and is visualized laparoscopically as a fibrous white tract. Its significance in hernia repair is that it forms superior boundary for the triangle of pain.

The spaces of the inguinal canal visualized by laparoscopy are divided into six groups: (1) superomedially by the space of Retzius, (2) superiorly by the space of Bogros, (3) laterally by the space of Dulucq, (4) inferomedially by the corona mortis, (5) inferiorly by the triangle of doom and (6) laterally by the triangle of pain.

Iliopectineal Arch

It is a thickened structure covering the iliac muscles and arches from anterior superior iliac spine inferiorly to the iliopubic eminence. It gives origin to portion of the internal oblique and transversus abdominis muscle as well as inguinal ligament.

Space of Retzius (Fig. 1.6)

This is the prevesical space that lies deep to the supravesical fossa and medial umbilical fossa and contains loose connective tissue. Fat dissection of the space is mandatory in a transabdominal preperitoneal (TAPP) or totally extraperitoneal (TEP) techniques to enable the medial border of the mesh to adequately overlap the medial edge of the defect.

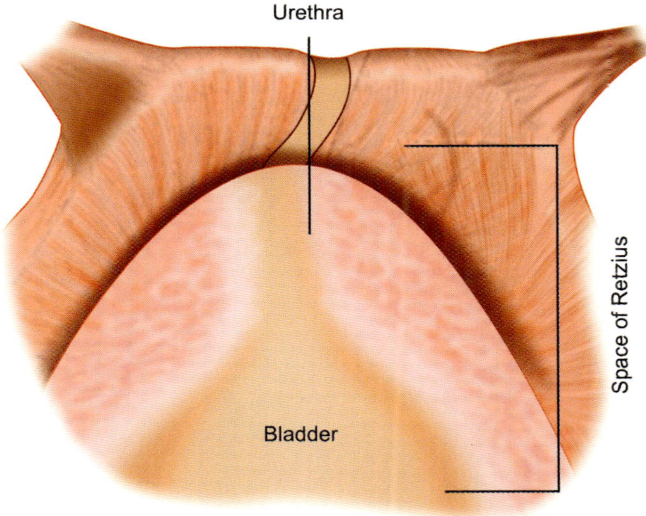

Fig. 1.6: Space of Retzius.

Important structures in this plane are:

- *Vascular*: External iliac artery and vein with its branches, i.e. deep circumflex iliac and inferior epigastric vessels.
- *Nerves*: Lateral femoral cutaneous nerve, genitofemoral, femoral, ilioinguinal, iliohypogastric and sympathetic plexus.
- *Lymphatics*: External iliac group of lymph nodes and associated deep lymphatics.
- Normal and aberrant obturator vessels.
- Accessory pudendal vessels (10%).

Space of Bogros

This is the preperitoneal space which actually forms the central aspect of the dissection under the peritoneum. This is continuous with the rectus space medially and continuous with Dulucq's space laterally. This is important because immediately anterior to the Bogros' space is the inferior epigastric artery and the deep ring.

Important structures in this space are indicated in Figure 1.7.

Dulucq's Space

This space continues as a lateral extension of the Bogros' space and extends laterally from the inferior epigastric artery right up to the iliopsoas below and lateral. Thus, from medial to lateral on the superior side, the surgeon while performing TAPP or TEP, will have to dissect the spaces of Retzius, Bogros and Dulucq in that order. We personally tend to dissect out the space

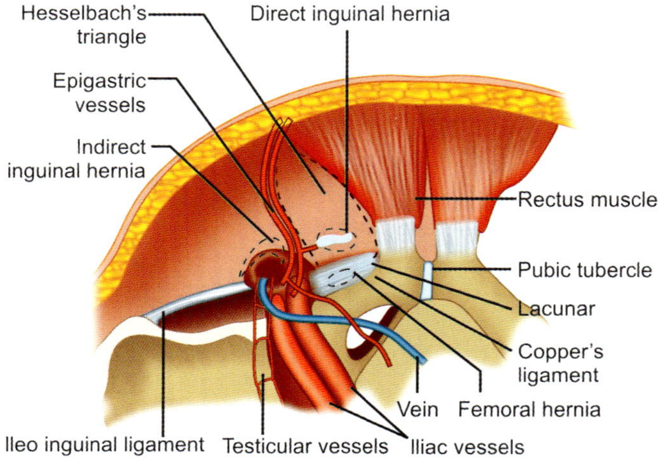

Fig. 1.7: Space of Bogros.

of Retzius first and then the space of Dulucq, and finally perform the dissection of the space of Bogros as the vital structures, namely the inferior epigastric artery, the vas and the testicular vessels run very close to this space.

Inferior epigastric artery is single, but the inferior epigastric vein is usually double, i.e. the two veins flank the inferior epigastric artery and joins the external iliac vein about 1 cm proximal to the inferior epigastric artery take off. Thus the inferior epigastric veins are a little more prone to injury than inferior epigastric artery. Some veins could pose a problem.

The deep venous circle of Bendavid is located in the space of Bogros as it is a circular network of deep inferior epigastric rectusial vein, retropubic and suprapubic veins. Care should be taken while dissecting out these small veins as hematoma could result in this situation.

OTHER VEINS

Iliopubic Vein

This vein courses deep into the iliopubic tract and joins the anterior pubic vein and could be injured dissecting out the iliopubic tract.

Rectorectal Vein of Bendavid

This vein runs along within the lower lateral fibers of the rectus and forms a venous anastomotic ring joining the iliopubic vein above the pubic crest.

Retropubic Vein

This vein is a small collateral branch of the anastomotic pubic vein and is observed on the inferior posterior aspect of the pubic ramus beneath the Cooper's ligament.

Corona Mortis (Fig. 1.8)

The pubic branch of the inferior epigastric artery courses in a vertical fashion inferiorly, crossing the Cooper's ligament and anastomosing with the obturator artery. In 25–30% of individuals (can be as high as 70–80%), the pubic branch is large and can replace the obturator artery. This large arterial branch (aberrant obturator artery) can partially encircle the neck of a hernia sac and be injured in a femoral hernia repair. It could also be injured while exposing the Cooper's ligament by freeing it of areolar adipose connective tissue. Because of this possibility an enlarged pubic branch of the inferior epigastric artery has in the past been known as the—"corona mortis". This danger of injury in this area is more significant of obturator veins.

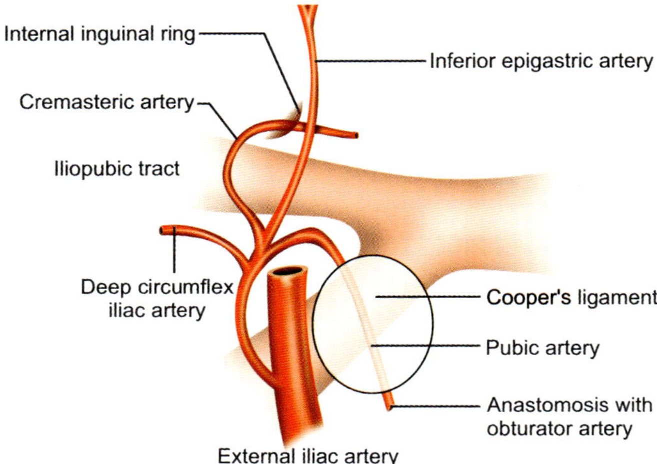

Fig. 1.8: Corona mortis.

What are the four nerves and the places where they are most easily injured? What will happen to them?

1. *Lateral femoral cutaneous nerve*: This nerve is the most commonly injured nerve during laparoscopic hernia repair.
   Course of the nerve: As it arises from L2-3, it emerges at the lateral edges of the psoas, and courses along the iliac fossa lateral to the iliac vessels. It passes below (or sometimes even through the fibers of) the inguinal ligament lying in a fibrous tunnel 1 cm medial to the anterior superior iliac spine. Its area of supply is the upper lateral aspect of thigh. Common site of injury in relation to the iliopubic tract is in the triangle of pain, resulting in the sequelae of pain and numbness in the upper lateral thigh called meralgia paresthetica or Bernhardt's syndrome.
2. *Genitofemoral nerve*: The femoral branch of the genital femoral nerve is at risk of damage during laparoscopic hernia repair. The genital branch of genitofemoral nerve is more often injured in an open inguinal repair. Sometimes if extensive maneuvers are performed to the sac and the perisac tissues at the internal ring, the genital branch of the genitofemoral nerve could be injured. Nerve arises from L1-2, courses through the psoas major occupying the anteromedial aspect of the muscle, dividing into genital and femoral branches before reaching the internal inguinal ring. The genital branch pierces the iliopubic tract lateral to the deep ring and then enters the ring (within 5 mm of the upper border of the ring, and courses through the inguinal canal). *This is the reason why when the peritoneum is opened in a TAPP; it is always opened at the point atleast 1 cm superior to the upper edge of the ring to avoid injury to the genital branch of the genital femoral nerve.* The femoral branch courses beneath

the inguinal ligament to the thigh. Area of supply of the genital branch is the cremaster, the spermatic fascia and tunica-vaginalis of the testes; it is also the efferent branch for the cremastric reflux, and in the female, it is sensory to the labium major. The femoral branch is the cutaneous branch to the skin over the femoral triangle and is the afferent branch for the cremasteric reflex.

Common site of the entrapment is on the posterior abdominal wall especially if tackers or staplers are used well below the iliopubic tract. Post injury, it causes pain in the groin, scrotum and upper thigh. Tenderness is found along the internal ring and along the inguinal canal with hyperextension or external rotation of the hip, thus increasing the pain. *The loss of cremasteric reflex indicates that either the genital, or the femoral branch or both have been injured during the operation.*

3. *Femoral nerve*: Usually the intermediate cutaneous branch of the anterior division of the femoral nerve is at risk during laparoscopic meshplasty although injury to the main trunk of the femoral nerve has also been described.

   Course of femoral nerve: Arising from L2-4, the femoral nerve emerges from the lateral aspect of the psoas muscle and travels, and courses below the inguinal ligament lateral to the femoral artery and outside the femoral sheath. Common site of injury is the posterior abdominal wall, well posterior to the ilioinguinal tract and little lateral to the genitofemoral nerve (medial to lateral are the genitofemoral nerve, the femoral nerve and then the lateral cutaneous nerve of the thigh). Post-injury pain could be the anteromedial aspect of the thigh with or without thigh paralgesia or paresthesia. Even a little hip extension causes pain. Later the quadriceps muscles weaken, and loss of patellar reflex could occur.
4. *Ilioinguinal nerve*: This nerve is rarely involved in laparoscopic hernia repair. It is frequently involved in open inguinal hernioplasty. It is only injured if excessive pressure is applied during laparoscopic mesh fixation, compressing the muscles sufficiently to allow the tacker or the stapler to reach the deeply situated nerve.

   Course of ilioinguinal nerve: Arising from L1, travels retroperitoneally across the quadratus lumborum behind the kidney and then passes anterior to the iliac muscles, piercing the transversus abdominis near the anterior end of the iliac crest, and then piercing the internal oblique. It travels through the inguinal canal in an anterolateral position in the spermatic cord and exits through the superficial inguinal ring or the external oblique aponeurosis.

   Area of supply:

- Skin at the root of the penis
- Anterior third of the scrotum

- Labium majora in female
- Small area of thigh inferomedial to the inguinal ligament
- Motor supply is the internal oblique before it reaches the inguinal canal.

  Common site of entrapment is medial to the anterosuperior iliac spine (only if excessive pressure is applied on the anterior abdominal wall during the mesh fixation).

  Post-injury paresthesia in the lower abdomen, scrotum and upper medial thigh. Extension of hip increases the pain.

Triangle of Doom (Fig. 1.9)

The boundaries of triangle of doom, medially it is vas deferens, laterally it is gonadal vessels and posteriorly it is peritoneal edge. The contents are the external iliac vessels, deep circumflex vein, femoral nerve and genital branch of genitofemoral nerve. The point to be remembered is that the mesh should not be fixed in this region to avoid "doom" bleeding complication.

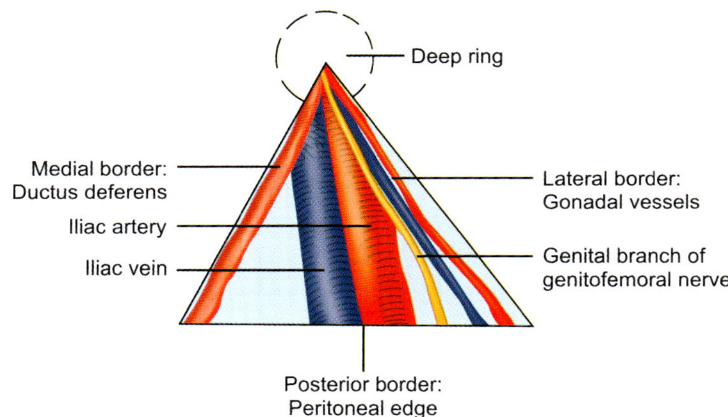

Fig. 1.9: Triangle of doom.

Triangle of Pain (Fig. 1.10)

The boundaries of triangle of pain are the spermatic cord medially, iliac crest laterally and superiorly the iliopubic tract. The contents, from lateral to medial, of triangle of pain are lateral femoral cutaneous nerve, anterior femoral cutaneous nerve, femoral branch of genitofemoral nerve and

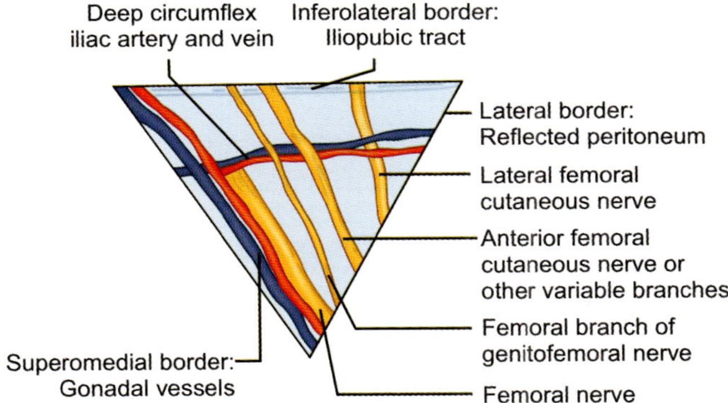

Fig. 1.10: Triangle of pain.

femoral nerve. The point to be remembered is electrocautery should not be used in this region. Dulucq's fascia covers these nerves and one should try not to strip off during dissection to avoid neuropraxia.

2

Total Extraperitoneal Repair

INDICATIONS

All inguinal hernias can be repaired by the total extraperitoneal (TEP) technique with the following exceptions:

- Irreducible hernias
- Large inguinoscrotal hernias
- Recurrent inguinal hernias after TEP or transabdominal preperitoneal (TAPP) technique (relative contraindications)
- Inguinal hernias and coexistent incisional or ventral hernia (TAPP technique is better in these circumstances).

POSITIONS

- Supine with contralateral arm abducted, and ipsilateral arm adducted and kept close to the body.
- Slight upward tilt of side of surgery.
- The surgeon stands between the abducted arm and the body, and the camera assistant stands between the contralateral shoulder and the abducted arm. The positions can be reversed if operating on bilateral hernias.

PRINCIPLE

The key step of this procedure is to access the preperitoneal space directly from above and to cover the complete posterior inguinal wall, exactly like in the TAPP repair, with an appropriate sized mesh.

MESH DETAILS

Material: Either polypropylene (light, medium or heavyweight), polyester or a composite mesh of polypropylene and poliglecaprone may be used in this space as there is no danger of contact with bowel.

Dimensions: A 15 cm × 12 cm size is most commonly preferred by surgeons all over the world and also by us. The smallest size acceptable is 15 cm × 10 cm.

Extent: The following four points of reference should be reached and covered by the concerned mesh:

1. Upper medial: The rectus muscle up to the midline and beyond.
2. Lower medial: The pubic symphysis and the contralateral pubic arch.
3. Upper lateral: The internal oblique and the transversus abdominis (inner surface).
4. Lower lateral: Iliopsoas muscle with the intact fascia of the same.

ANESTHESIA

We find that spinal anesthesia is adequate for the TEP repair most of the time. Rarely, especially if the peritoneum is breached, conversion to general anesthesia may be required.

TECHNICAL STEPS

This procedure is broadly divided into four steps:

1. Creation and expansion of the preperitoneal plane
2. Dissection and exposure of the structures in the posterior inguinal wall
3. Dealing with the direct or indirect sac
4. Deployment of the mesh.

Creation of the Preperitoneal Plane

A transverse subumbilical incision (Fig. 2.1) is made on the midline on the skin, Camper's and Scarpa's fascias until the white and glistening anterior rectus sheath is reached (Fig. 2.2).

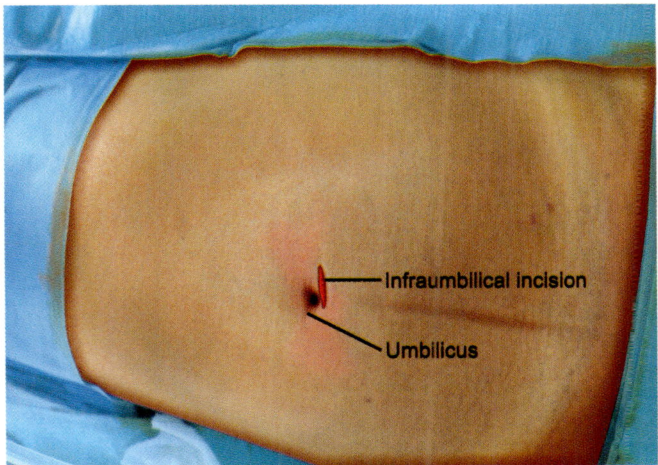

Fig. 2.1: Infraumbilical incision.

The S-shaped retractors are inserted into this 12 mm incision, and the anterior rectus sheath (Fig. 2.3) is cut transversely to expose the muscle underneath.

A pair of Allis forceps is used to catch the upper and lower edges of the sheath. The underlying rectus muscle is pulled laterally with the S-shaped retractor so as to expose the posterior rectus sheath.

The Allis forceps holding the upper edge is released and the Allis forceps holding the lower edge is retracted upward. This exposes the plane of the posterior rectus sheath clearly.

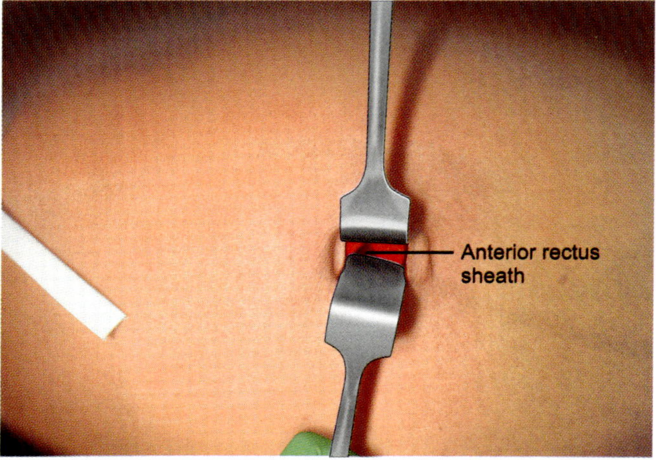

Fig. 2.2: Seeing the anterior rectus sheath.

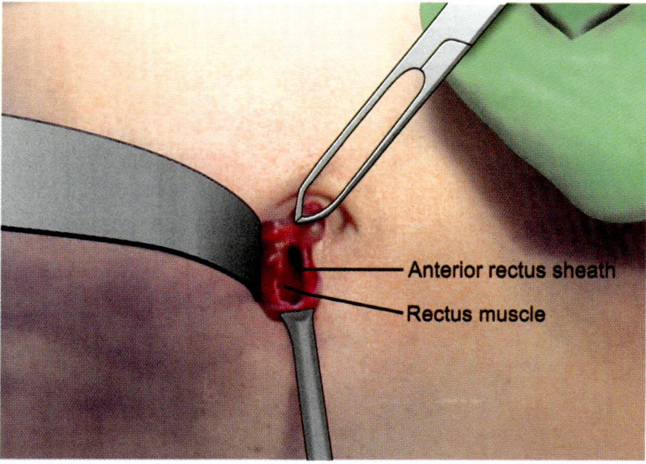

Fig. 2.3: Transverse incision on anterior rectus sheath.

The 2-0 polyglactin-910 (Vicryl) suture is used and a purse string is taken to include the cut edges of the sheath. A 10 mm cannula (Fig. 2.4) is inserted in this plane without the trocar and the purse string suture is tied (Fig. 2.5).

Dissection and Exposure of the Structures in the Posterior Inguinal Wall

The skin edges are grasped with towel clips or sutured to prevent CO_2 leak.

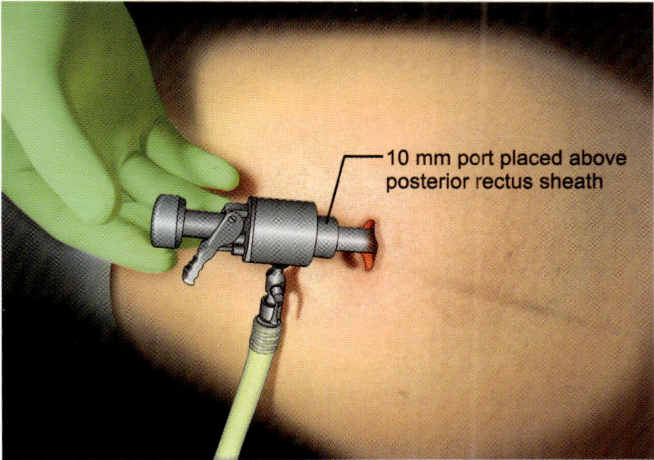

Fig. 2.4: Port placed above posterior rectus sheath.

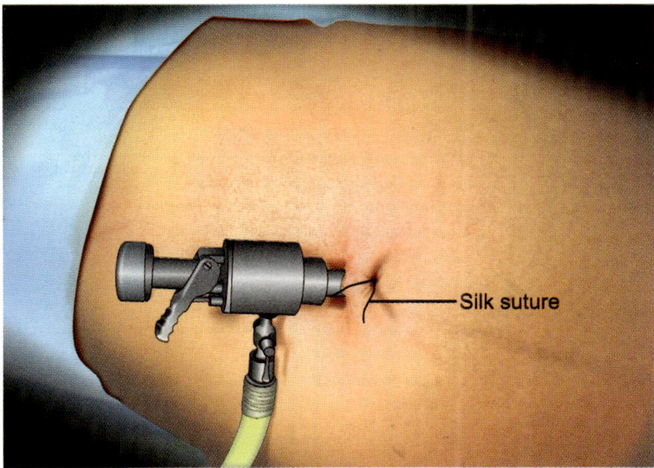

Fig. 2.5: Skin sutured to prevent gas leak.

A high-pressure CO_2 insufflation is done (16–20 mm). This permits expansion and capno dissection of the preperitoneal space. Even a balloon as seen in Figure 2.6 can be used to create preperitoneal space.

With a 0° telescope, the preperitoneal space is inspected, and with gentle to and fro and side-to-side movements, the space is developed toward the ipsilateral pubic bone (Fig. 2.7). When this space is reached, the white shining periosteum of the pubic bone is seen, and this is known as "the lighthouse sign" (Fig. 2.8).

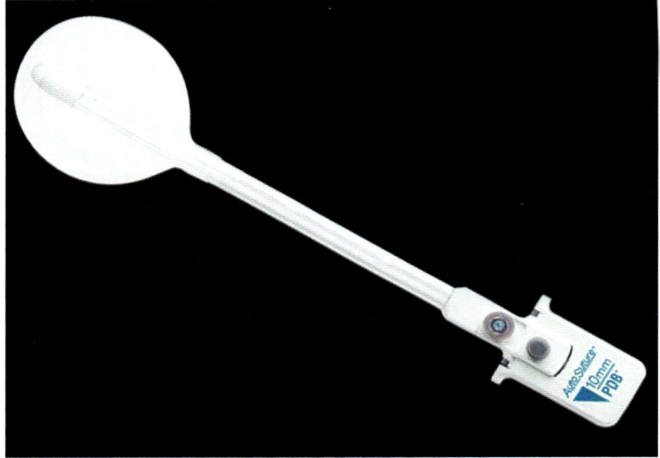

Fig. 2.6: Balloon used for creating preperitoneal space.

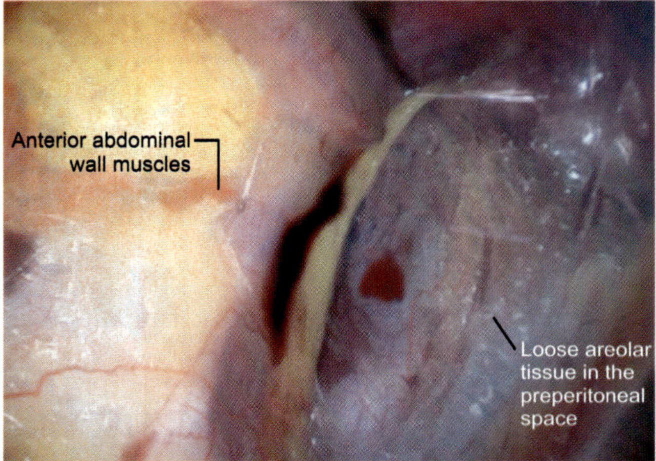

Fig. 2.7: Preperitoneal space.

Gentle dissection is continued laterally from the lighthouse toward the posterior wall of the inguinal canal. Dissection is also commenced beyond the midline so as to visualize the contralateral ramus.

Now the 0° telescope is exchanged for a 30° telescope—one looking upward at the anterior wall. This exposes the inferior epigastric artery clearly, and the inner surface of the rectus muscle is well displayed in the midline. Any direct defect will be seen immediately as preperitoneal space is created in midline (Fig. 2.9).

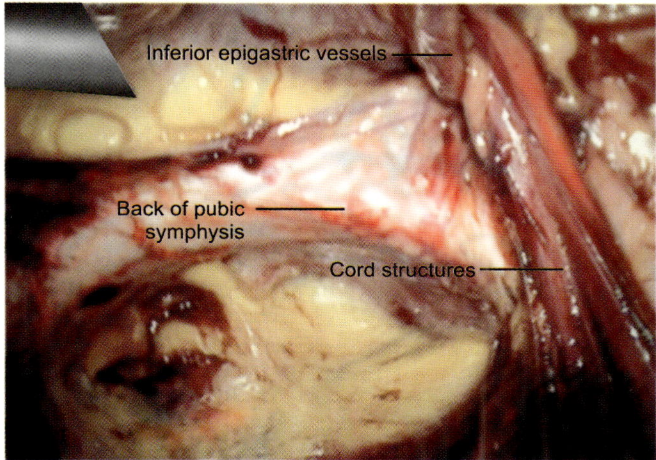

Fig. 2.8: Lighthouse sign.

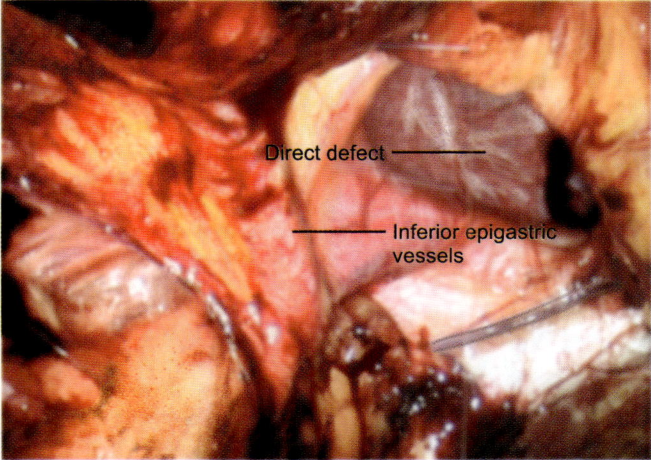

Fig. 2.9: Direct defect seen.

At this point, the second port is inserted in the suprapubic area, and this is followed by the third port midway between the suprapubic and the subumbilical ports. Both these ports are 5 mm ports.

Blunt nosed, non-toothed straight graspers are inserted into both 5 mm or working ports, and the preperitoneal space is expanded and dissected by a series of spreading movements with one grasper elevating the anterior abdominal wall and the other holding back the peritoneum and the posterior wall tissues.

Further medial dissection exposes the pubic symphysis and the retropubic space with the bladder seeming to be in a deeper plane. The obturator foramen is dissected and the obturator internus muscle is seen, and the obturator nerve and vessels are visualized; this marks the inferior limit of the dissection.

Now the attention is turned to the dissection of the inguinal canal. For this, the approach is by going deep to the inferior epigastric artery and toward the anterior superior iliac spine. The cobweb-like fascia (Dulucq's fascia) is dissected until the iliopsoas fascia is seen with the underlying nerves—genital and femoral branches of the genitofemoral nerve, main femoral nerve and the lateral cutaneous nerve of thigh—from medial to lateral (Fig. 2.10).

Dealing with the Direct or Indirect Sac

After the medial and lateral dissection of the extraperitoneal space, attention is turned to the central part in relation to the inferior epigastric artery.

The relation of the sac to inferior epigastric artery is now ascertained. If a direct sac is found, it is dissected posteriorly and the pseudo sac is pushed anteriorly as described in the TAPP. An indirect sac is found by splaying the structures lateral and inferior to the inferior epigastric artery (Fig. 2.11). It is dealt

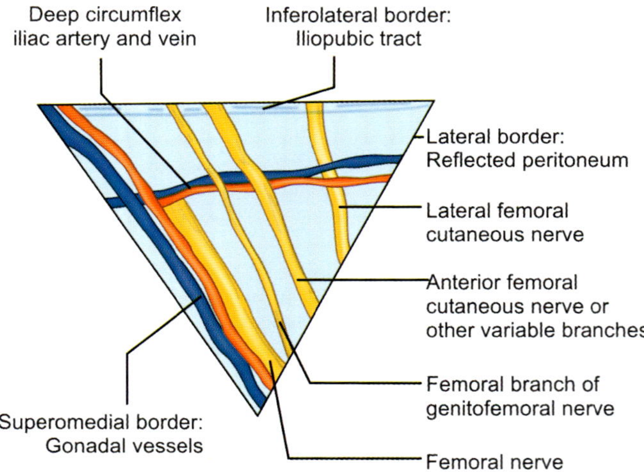

Fig. 2.10: Triangle of pain.

with by traction dissection and posterior reduction (if easy) (Fig. 2.12) or by cutting across the sac and applying a purse string suture (if difficult) (Figs. 2.13 and 2.14). As the medial, lateral and central parts of the dissection are joined together, the posterior wall of the canal is widely exposed.

Deployment of the Mesh

The peritoneal edge should be pushed back well away from the internal ring up to a point of wide divergence of the vas from the testicular vessels.

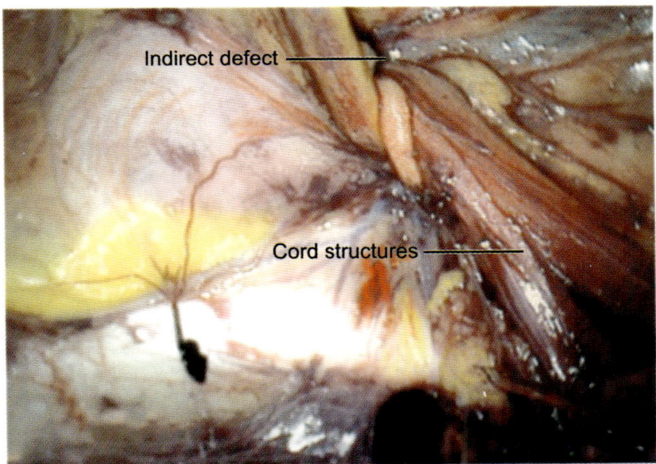

Fig. 2.11: Indirect defect.

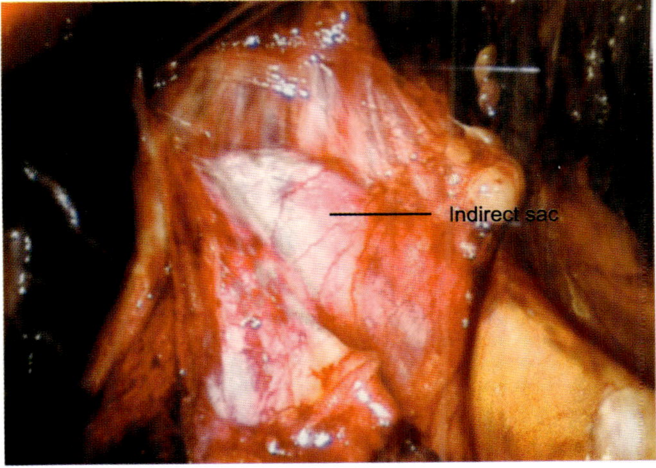

Fig. 2.12: Indirect sac dissection.

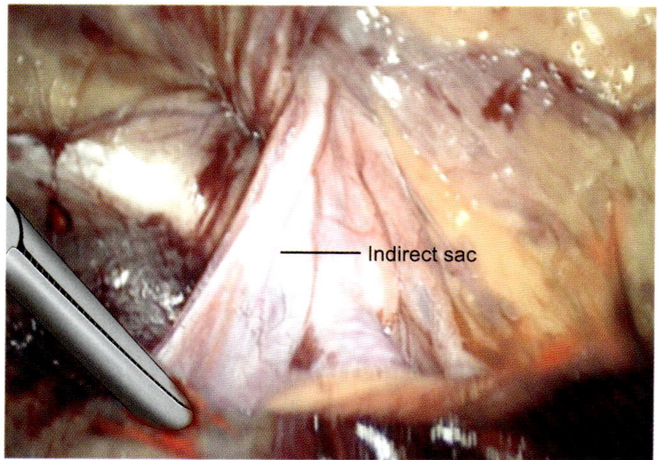

Fig. 2.13: Indirect sac dissection.

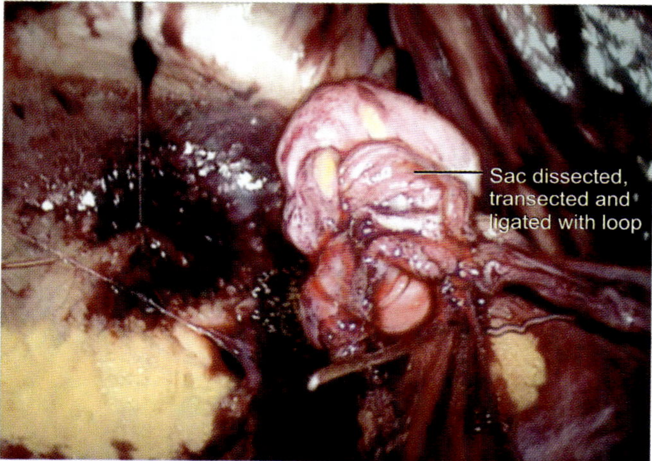

Fig. 2.14: Sac ligated with loop.

A 15 cm × 12 cm mesh is cut and rolled (Fig. 2.15), and backloaded into the optical cannula (Fig. 2.16). The mesh is grasped and orientated exactly as described in chapter 3 "Transabdominal Preperitoneal Repair". The mesh is unrolled and spread out to cover myopectineal orifice of Fruchaud (Fig. 2.17).

Unlike the TAPP, the TEP does not necessarily require the fixation of the mesh (Fig. 2.18). This potential space effectively closes up after desufflation. However, if the defect is wide or recurrent, we use two tacks, one into the Cooper's ligament (Fig. 2.19) and one medial to inferior epigastric artery along the upper edge.

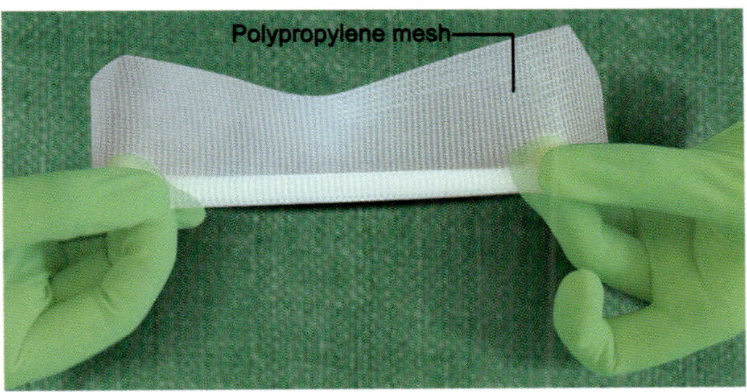

Fig. 2.15: Prolene mesh used in TEP.

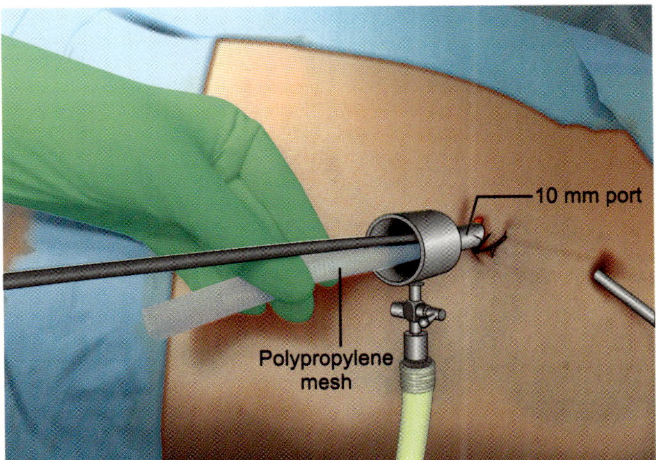

Fig. 2.16: Introduction of polypropylene mesh.

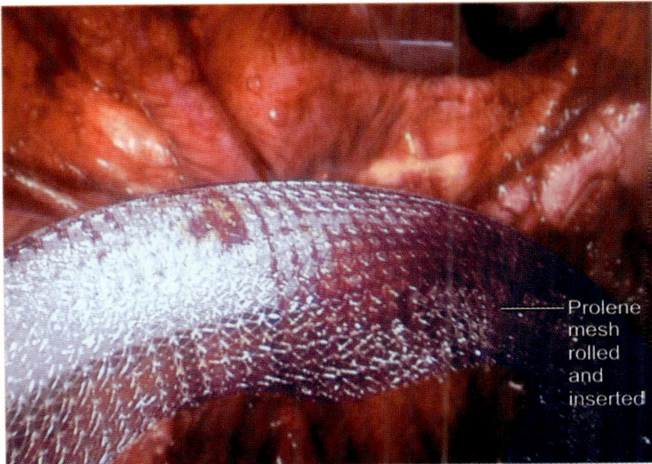

Fig. 2.17: Mesh inserted.

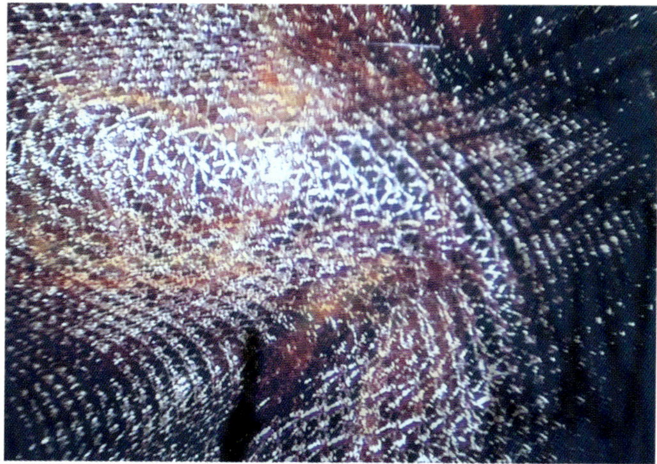

Fig. 2.18: Mesh placed in preperitoneal space.

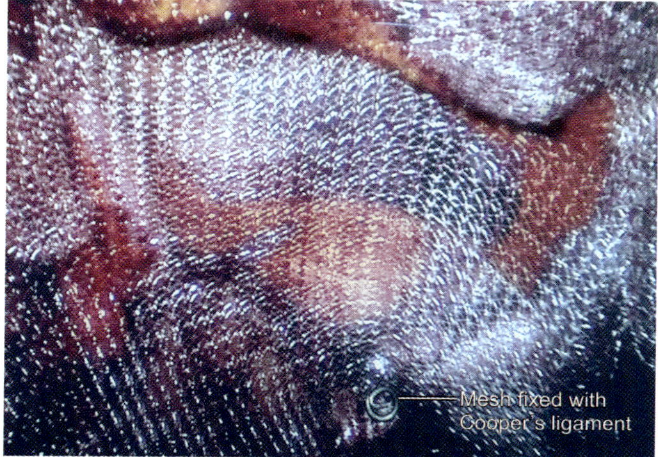

Fig. 2.19: Mesh fixed with Cooper's ligament.

With the mesh being held down onto the iliac vessels and with the peritoneal edge being seen well behind the mesh, the space is desufflated. This is an important step to prevent the peritoneum from rolling between the mesh and anterior wall.

The cannulae are removed and the sheath closed with 2-0 polyglactin-910 suture and the skin closed with the 3-0 poliglecaprone (Monocryl) suture.

Chapter

3

Transabdominal Preperitoneal Prosthesis

Transabdominal preperitoneal prosthesis (TAPP) which indicates entry into the preperitoneal space through the abdominal cavity.

INDICATIONS

- All direct and indirect inguinal hernias can be repaired with this technique.
- It is preferred over the total extraperitoneal prosthesis (TEP) in the case of large indirect inguinal hernias and irreducible inguinal hernias.
- Patients who are undergoing another intraperitoneal procedure, such as ovarian cystectomy, splenectomy, etc. can have a TAPP if they also have an inguinal hernia.

We recommend that surgeons starting laparoscopic inguinal hernia repair may begin with the TAPP technique, which permitting familiarization with the complex inguinal anatomy, before proceeding to the TEP type of repair.

PRINCIPLE

The anchor of the TAPP procedure is the access to the preperitoneal plane from the peritoneal cavity. This is the same plane that has been described in chapter 2 "Total Extraperitoneal Repair". Once this plane has been reached and widely dissected out, deployment of the mesh is done to cover the posterior inguinal wall completely.

MESH DETAILS

Discussed in chapter 2 "Total Extraperitoneal Repair".

TECHNICAL DETAILS

Anesthesia: Unlike the TEP technique, this procedure is always performed under general anesthesia as it always entails a pneumoperitoneum.
Position: Supine with both the arms abducted to 90°.

We use a standard Veress needle to initiate pneumoperitoneum and insufflate an initial 2 L of carbon dioxide.

The first port (11 mm) is inserted immediately below the umbilicus through a vertical or transverse cut. This is the optical port.

A 10 mm 30° telescope is inserted through the optic port. The telescope faces upward, i.e. to look up at the anterior abdominal wall (Fig. 3.1).

The next two ports are along the right and left midclavicular lines 1 cm below the level of the optical port so as to form a gentle optical triangle. Both these ports are 5 mm (Fig. 3.2).

The patient is tilted into the head down position with a rotation so as to bring the side of surgery above, e.g. right up position for a right inguinal

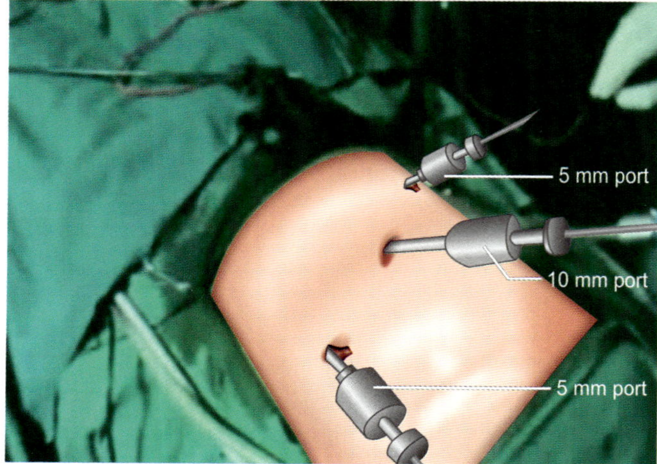

Fig. 3.1: Port placement for left inguinal hernia repair.

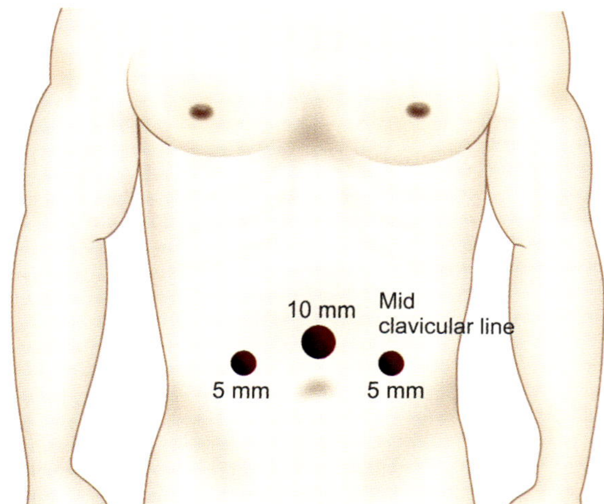

Fig. 3.2: Port placement for bilateral TAPP.

hernia. A Maryland's forceps is inserted into the left 5 mm port and an L-hook is inserted into the right port (the rest of the description continues for a right inguinal hernia) (Fig. 3.3).

At this point, the anatomy of the inguinal canal is noted:

- In the midline, the median umbilical ligament runs from the apex of the bladder to the umbilicus (contains the obliterated urachus). Further laterally, the medial umbilical ligament runs at the apex of a peritoneal fold from the medial aspect of the inguinal canal up to the umbilicus carrying the obliterated umbilical artery. Still more laterally, the lateral umbilical ligament is the fold of peritoneum that is raised by the inferior epigastric artery and vein (Fig. 3.4).
- At the lower end of the lateral umbilical ligament, the deep inguinal ring is found into which the testicular vessels run from the lateral side and the vas deferens runs in from the medial side (Fig. 3.5).

The triangle between the vas deferens and the testicular vessels is known as the "triangle of doom", and it refers to the underlying iliac artery and vein.

The iliopubic tract is a thickened band of tendinous fascia that runs from the anterior superior iliac spine to the pubic tubercle. The triangle between the peritoneal edge, the testicular vessels and the iliopubic tract is known as the "triangle of pain" as it houses four nerves that run on the iliopsoas, viz. the lateral cutaneous nerve of thigh, the femoral nerve and the femoral and genital branches of the genitofemoral nerve, from lateral to medial.

The corona mortis or "the circle of death" refers to the anastomotic network between the pubic branch of the cremasteric vessels and the pubic branch of the obturator. These vessels run on the posterior aspect of the pubic ramus and on Cooper's ligament.

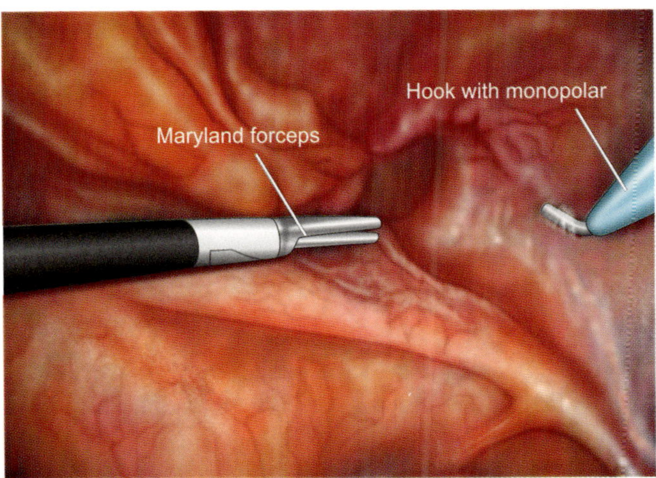

Fig. 3.3: Opening the peritoneum with monopolar hook.

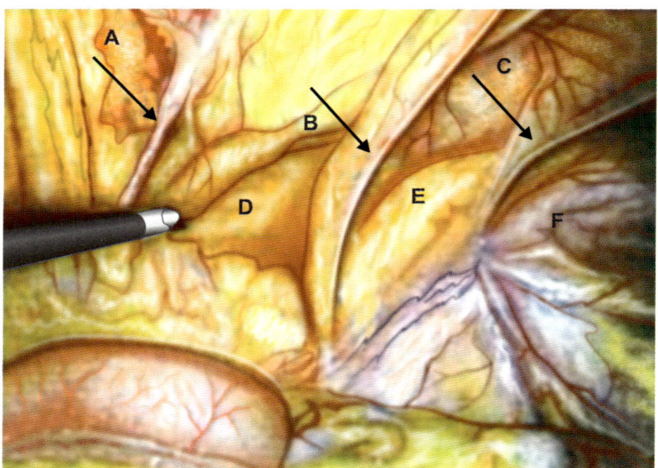

Fig. 3.4: Laparosopic view of normal pelvic anatomy on the right side (before peritoneal reflection).
Keys: A, median umbilical ligament; B, medial umbilical ligament; C, lateral umbilical ligament; D, supravesical fossa; E, medial fossa; F, lateral fossa.

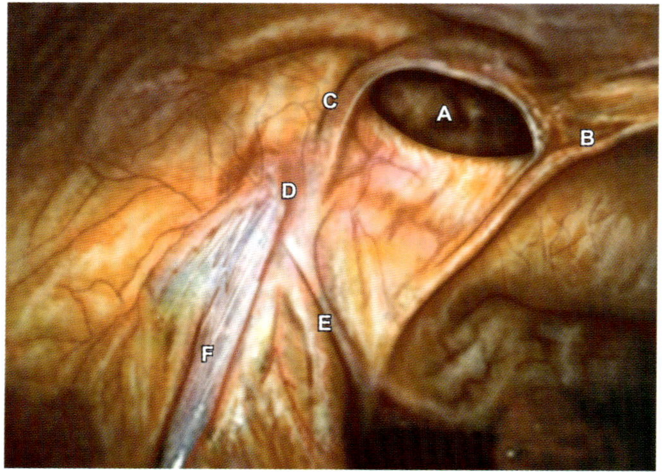

Fig. 3.5: Left direct hernia before peritoneal reflection.
Keys: A, direct defect; B, medial umbilical ligament; C, lateral umbilical ligament; D, internal ring; E, vas deference; F, spermatic vessels.

The Cooper's ligament is a thick tendinous structure running from the pubic tubercle posteriorly and parallel to the iliopubic tract. This offers the best place to fix the mesh inferomedially.

With the Maryland's forceps lifting up the peritoneum, the L-hook faces forward and a gentle diathermy burn is made to cut open the peritoneum

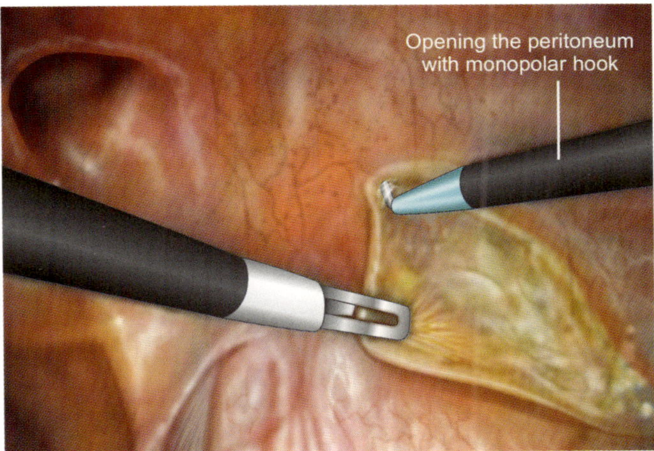

Fig. 3.6: Capno-dissection.

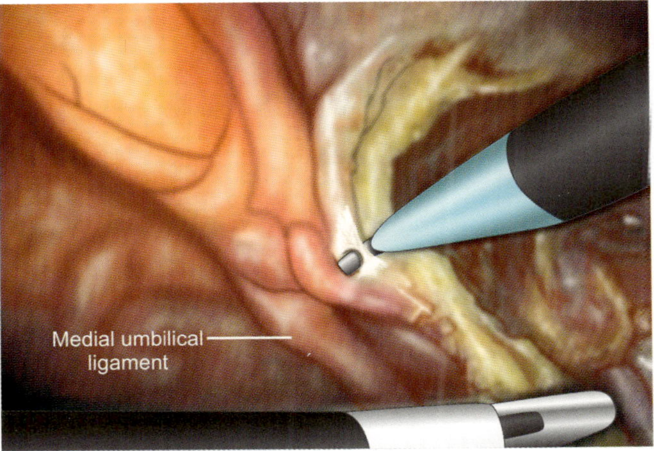

Fig. 3.7: Opening peritoneum till medial umbilical ligament.

at a point 2 cm medial and 2 cm inferior to the anterior superior iliac spine. The burn is made after the point is confirmed by external palpation (Fig. 3.6).

After the peritoneum is opened, the pneumoperitoneum is permitted to enter the subperitoneal space (capno-dissection).

The hook is inserted into the space facing medially, and the peritoneal edge is cut from lateral to medial, skirting the deep inguinal ring by at least 5 mm (in order to avoid the genital branch of the genitofemoral nerve).

The peritoneal cut is taken across and superficial to the inferior epigastric vessels (the lateral umbilical ligament), and further medially until the medial umbilical ligament is reached (Fig. 3.7).

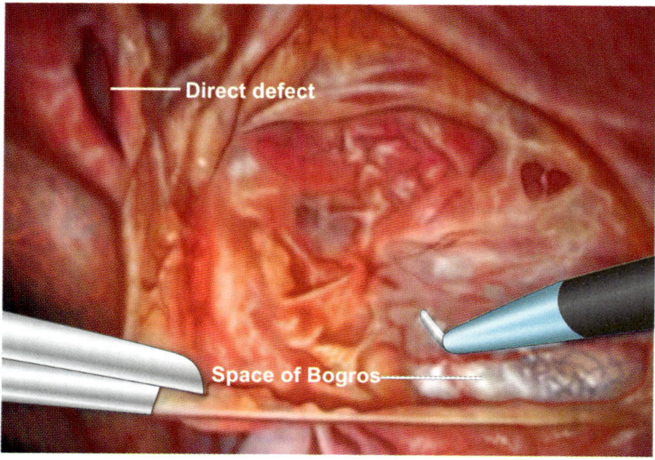

Fig. 3.8: Reflecting the peritoneum.

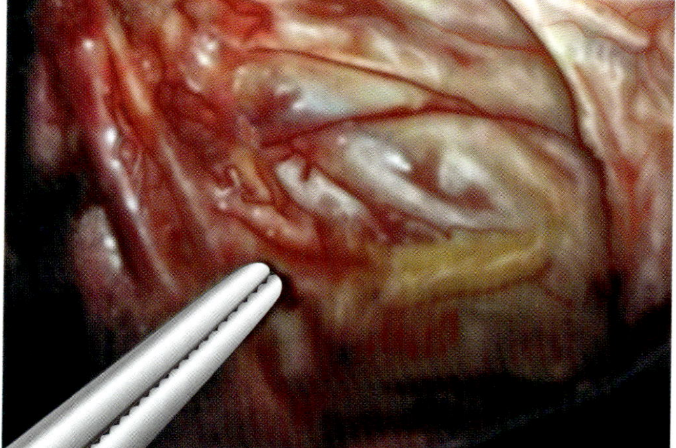

Fig. 3.9: Space of Bogros.

The lower edge of the peritoneal flap is grasped with the Maryland's forceps and the flap is raised, pushing aside the testicular vessels, which will be seen in the lateral aspect of the flap. The object of the dissection is to hold onto the peritoneum alone and to parietalize all other structures (Fig. 3.8).

In the lateral aspect of the dissection, the iliopsoas muscle with its overlying fascia is seen. The nerves run deep to the fascia and on the surface of the muscles. It is important not to dissect out the fascia and expose the nerves otherwise the mesh may get adherent to the nerves and cause chronic pain. Attention is then given to the medial aspect of the dissection

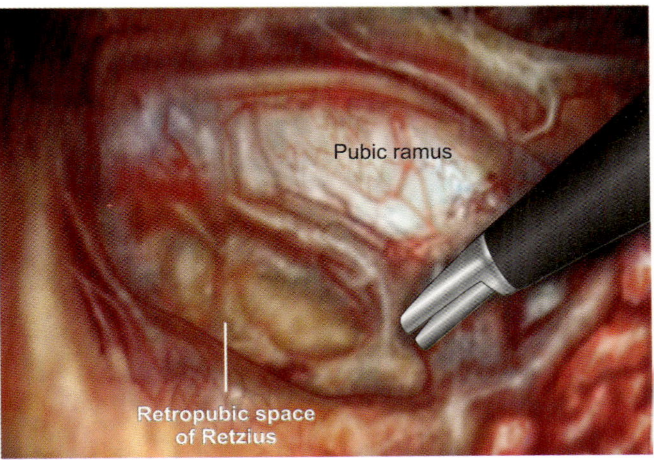

Fig. 3.10: Space of Retzius.

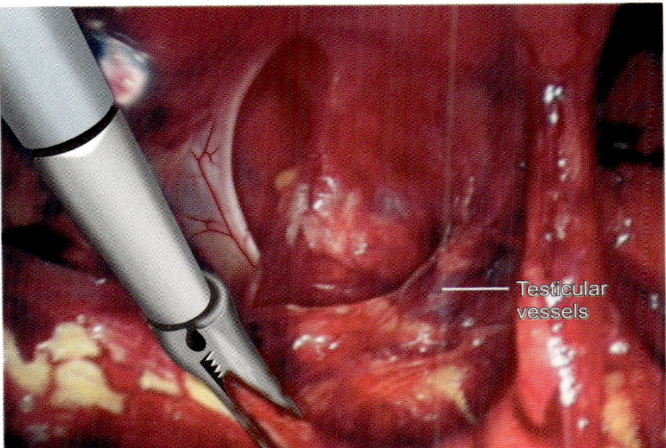

Fig. 3.11: Dissection of cord structures.

(Fig. 3.9). If the peritoneal cut extends too medially up to the median umbilical ligament, there is a danger of damage to the bladder.

The dissection is deepened under the medial umbilical ligament until the glistening white periosteum of the pubic ramus is seen (Fig. 3.10).

Now the peritoneal area between the medial and lateral dissection is extended and the direct or indirect sac will be dealt with accordingly.

Direct sac: If a direct sac is found (medial to the inferior epigastric vessels), the peritoneal cut is extended above the upper border of the sac to join the medial dissection (Figs. 3.11 and 3.12).

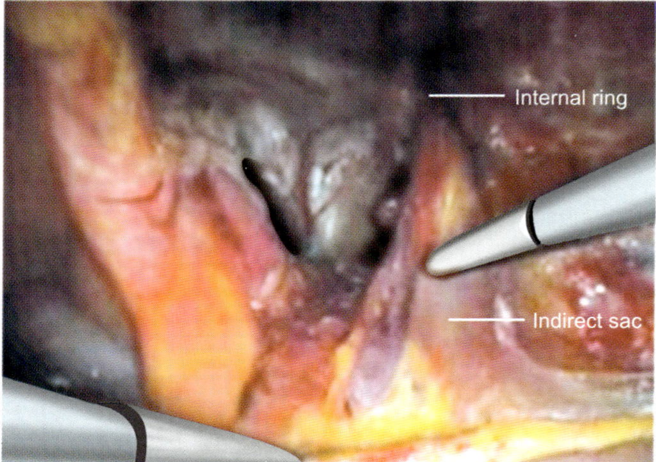

Fig. 3.12: Dissecting indirect hernia.

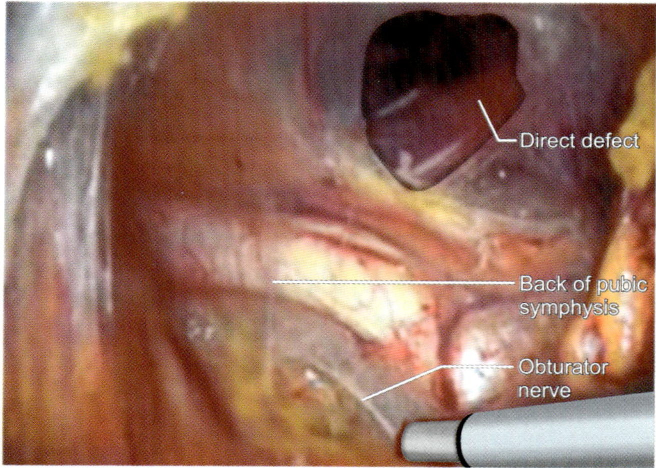

Fig. 3.13: Obturator nerve.

Then the sac edge is grasped with the Maryland's forceps and, with gentle hook dissection, the peritoneum is peeled off the defect, thus exposing the pseudo sac underneath (Fig. 3.13).

The pseudo sac is allowed to go anteriorly to the defect. Some workers tack the pseudo sac to the Cooper's ligament in order to lessen the incidence of seroma. But, we leave the pseudo sac alone.

Indirect sac: Indirect sac is seen entering the inguinal canal lateral to the inferior epigastric vessels and through the deep ring. This is dealt with in one of two ways: the cut edge of the peritoneum is held with the Maryland's

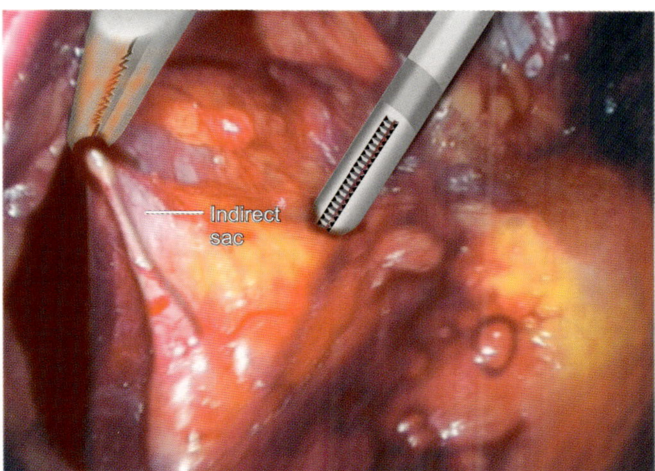

Fig. 3.14: Indirect sac.

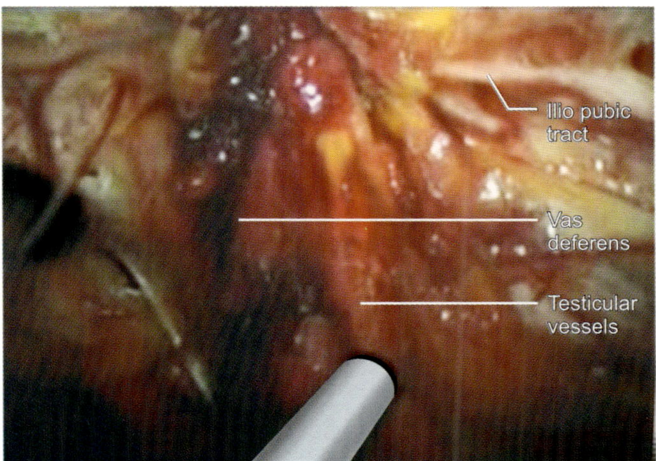

Fig. 3.15: Testicular vessels.

forceps and traction is given to deliver the sac proximally (Figs. 3.14 and 3.15). This is done after any contents are reduced.

The other technique is to extend the peritoneal cut across the sac and leave the distal portion inside the canal.

The last important step before mesh deployment is to parietalize the cord structures. This is done by peeling off the lower edge of the peritoneum from the underlying vas and testicular vessels (Fig. 3.16).

This parietalization should proceed for a distance of at least 5–6 cm from the edge of the internal ring or at least until the vas and testicular vessels are found to diverge from each other (Fig. 3.17).

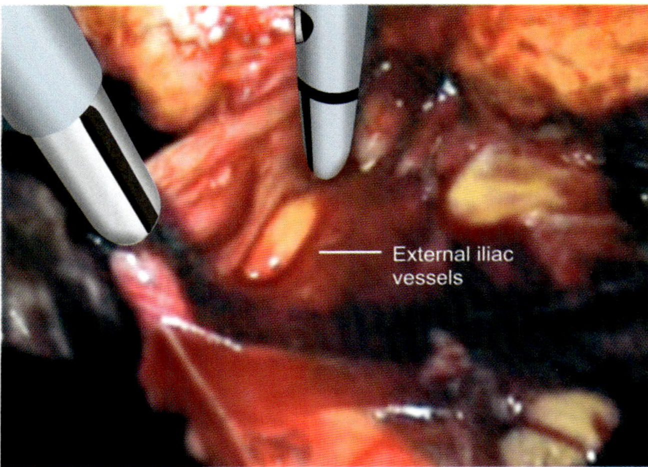

Fig. 3.16: External illiac vessels.

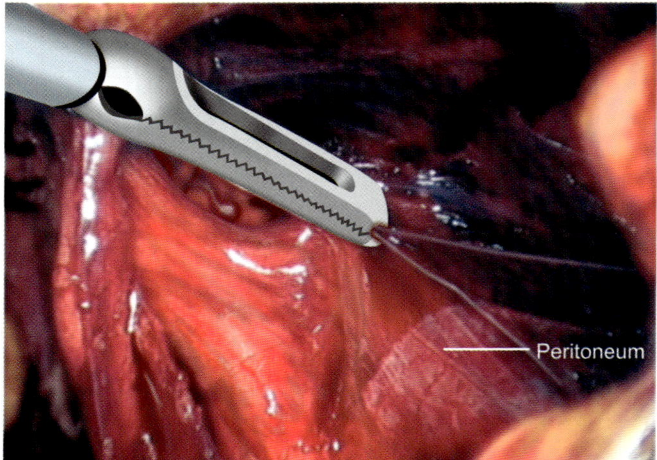

Fig. 3.17: Peritoneum reflected back.

The parietalization is complete when the entire posterior wall structures are exposed.

Now the mesh is cut to a 15 cm × 12 cm size, rolled and taken in with a new toothed grasping forceps through the 10 mm port (Fig. 3.18).

It is then held and aligned so that the lower medial portion is tucked under the medial umbilical ligament. This edge is preferably rounded off with the scissors to avoid possible prostate irritation postoperatively (Fig. 3.19).

As the lower medial edge is tucked in along the pubic ramus, the upper edge is held up to the rectus muscle and a 5 mm tacker device is deployed

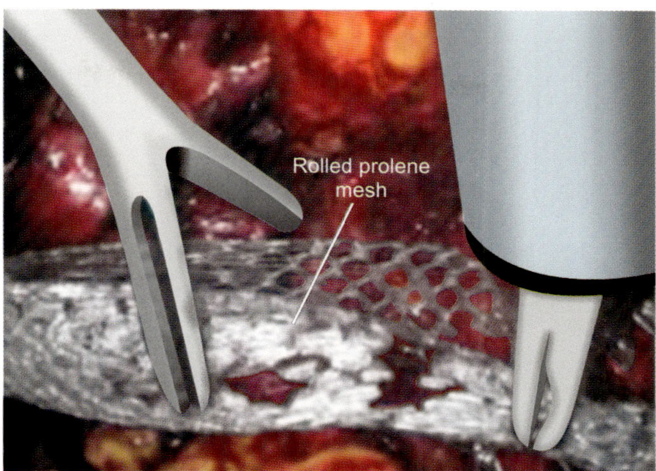

Fig. 3.18: Mesh introduction.

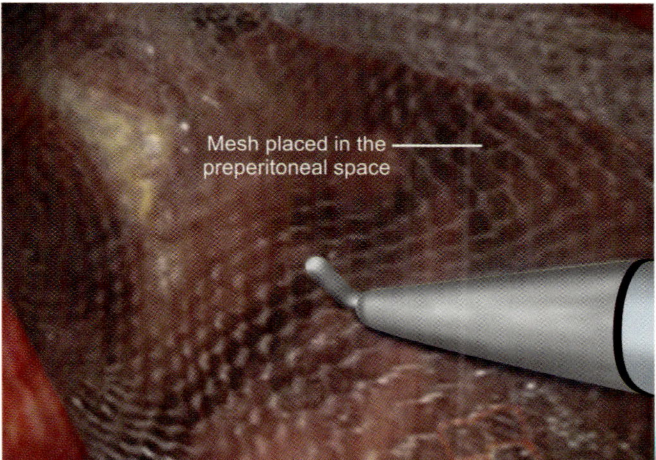

Fig. 3.19: Light weight prolene mesh placed in the preperitoneal plane.

to fix the superomedial and the inferomedial corners of the mesh with the rectus muscle and the Cooper's ligament respectively (Fig. 3.20).

The tacker is used to palpate the bone medially and is then displaced laterally until the yielding feel of the Cooper's ligament is reached. Care is taken to avoid any of the vessels of the corona mortis in this area.

The superolateral corner of the mesh is tacked against the body wall muscles laterally just below and medial to the anterior superior iliac spine.

The inferolateral corner of the mesh is not tacked, but only smoothed over the iliopsoas fascia.

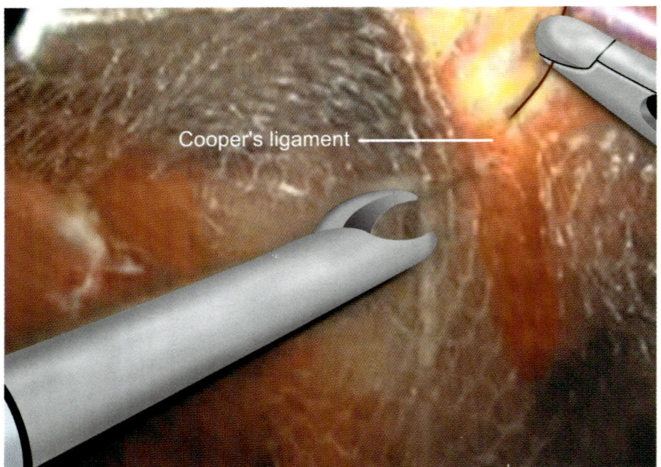

Fig. 3.20: Mesh sutured to Cooper's ligament.

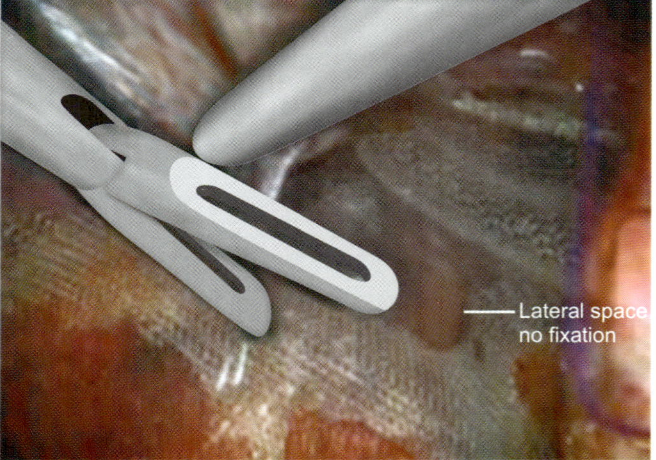

Fig. 3.21: Mesh in the lateral space.

The upper and lower edges of the mesh are tucked under the corresponding peritoneal flaps.

A 25 cm 2-0 polypropylene suture is back loaded into a 10-5 mm reducer and then inserted through the subumbilical cannula into the peritoneal cavity. Curved needle holders are inserted into the right and left working ports (Fig. 3.21).

The needle is grasped and the first suture is performed at the medial end of the peritoneal incision. The suture is completed and the peritoneal flap approximated from medial to lateral (toward the suturing instrument) by a series of running bites (Fig. 3.22).

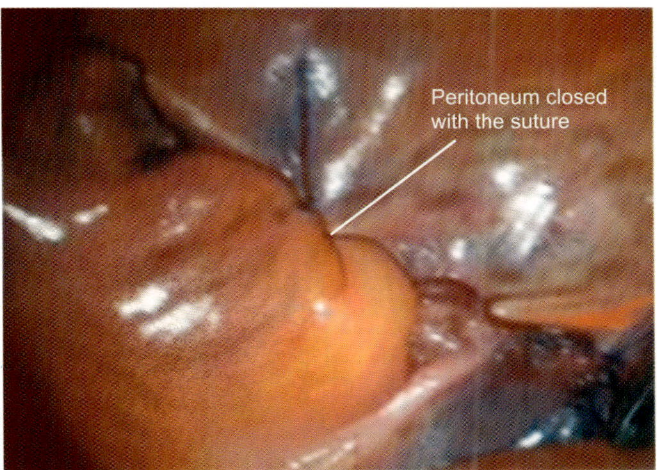

Fig. 3.22: Peritoneum closed with the suture.

As the suturing is done, the intraperitoneal pressure is dropped to facilitate peritoneal approximation (from 12 mm down to 9 mm).

One must be careful not to include the underlying mesh in the suture line as this would unroll the mesh and cause a recurrence. The suture is completed laterally and is cut with the scissors from the left hand working port.

The needle and suture are removed along with the cannula of the right hand working port.

Pneumoperitoneum is desufflated, the ports closed with 2-0 polyglactin 910 and the skin closed with 3-0 poliglecaprone.

Chapter

4

Decision Making—Open or Laparoscopic Ventral Hernia Mesh Plasty

INTRODUCTION

The following points are based both on the last 18 years of experience at our institution (JSR) and also based on the large volume of data published across the world.

When a patient has a flabby lower abdominal wall (Fig. 4.1), with a significant overhang (fatty apron), and wishes to have a cosmetically appealing and flat belly then such a candidate is an ideal one for an abdominoplasty—tummy tuck procedure in which the entire apron is excised after creating a cutaneous flap from the pubis all the way up to both costal margins (Figs. 4.2 to 4.4). The patient should be told that the surgery involves a long suprapubic incision from anterior superior iliac spine to anterior superior iliac spine (ASIS to ASIS) and a flap raised up to both costal margins, with a large dead space and a considerable possible drainage for a few days (Fig. 4.6). Hospital stay for 3–7 days is the rule after this operation. The umbilicus can either be preserved or resited at an appropriate position or a neoumbilicus can be formed (Fig. 4.5).

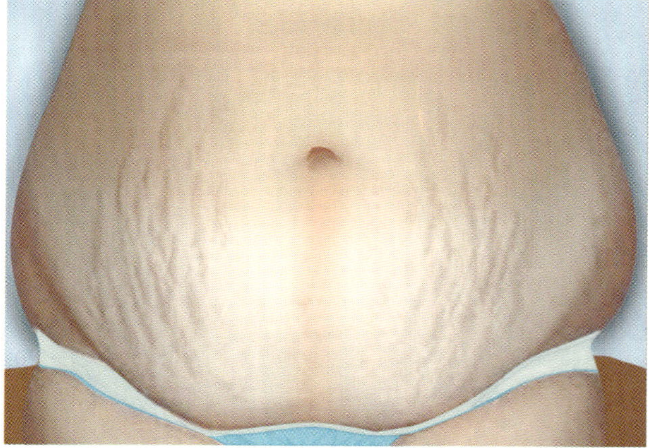

Fig. 4.1: Flabby abdomen.

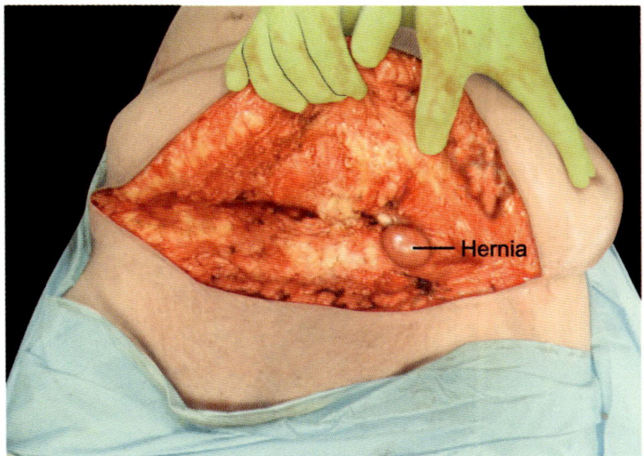

Fig. 4.2: Flap raising in abdominoplasty.

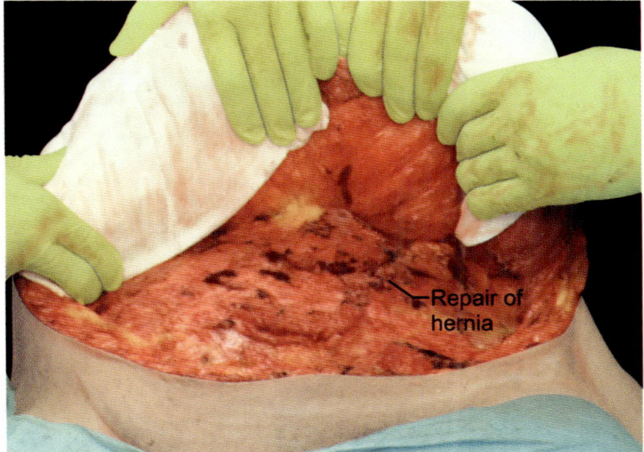

Fig. 4.3: Repair of hernia.

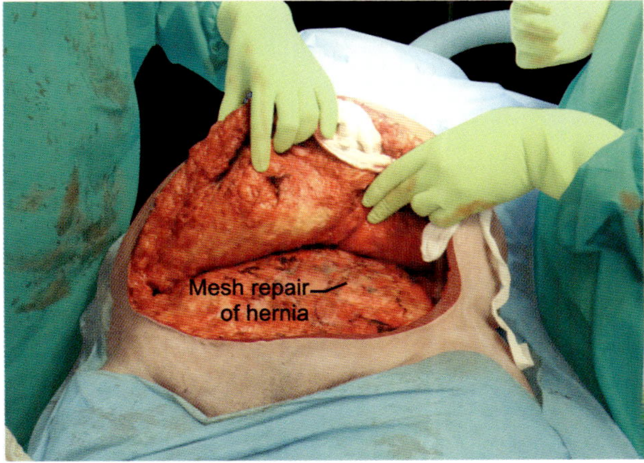

Fig. 4.4: Mesh repair.

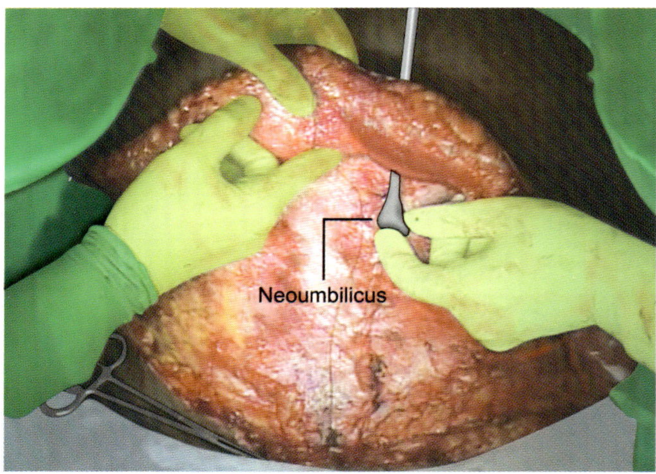

Fig. 4.5: Neoumbilicus.

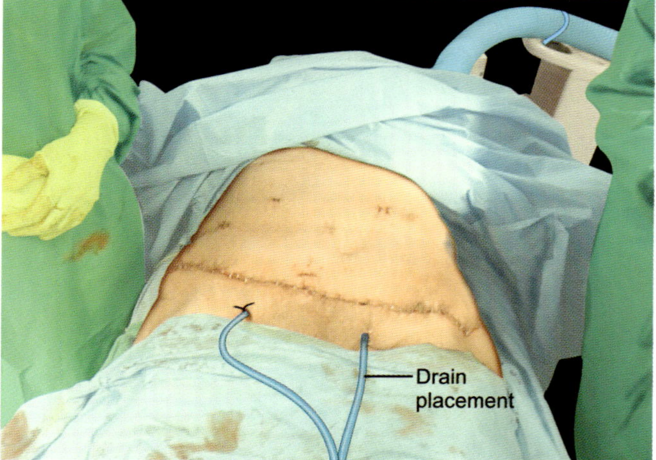

Fig. 4.6: Drain placement.

The surface area of the ventral hernia is measured. Most ventral hernias are truncated ellipses. If tangential lines are drawn along the vertical and horizontal edges of the ellipse a rectangle is found which is known as rectangle of fascial weakness. The older repairs of suturing the mesh only to the edge of the defect had a failure rate accountable by weakness of the neighboring fascia and therefore fascial weakness are looked at as rectangles to diminish recurrence (Fig. 4.7).

The surface area of the anterior abdominal wall is then calculated. The xiphopubic line is measured (from the xiphoid process to the pubic symphysis) and the interspinous line is also drawn (ASIS to ASIS); a vertical

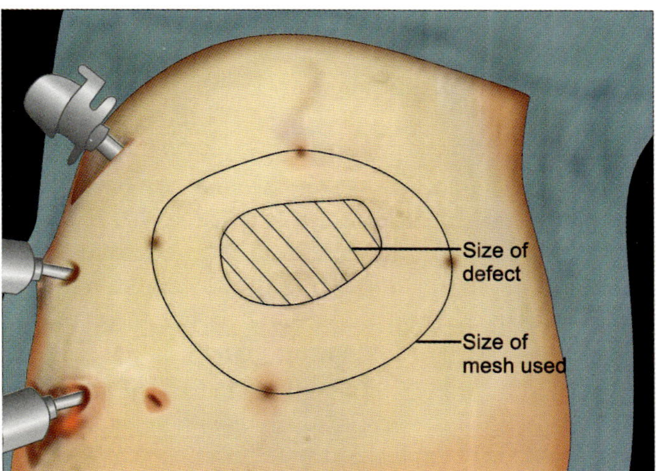

Fig. 4.7: Measurement of mesh.

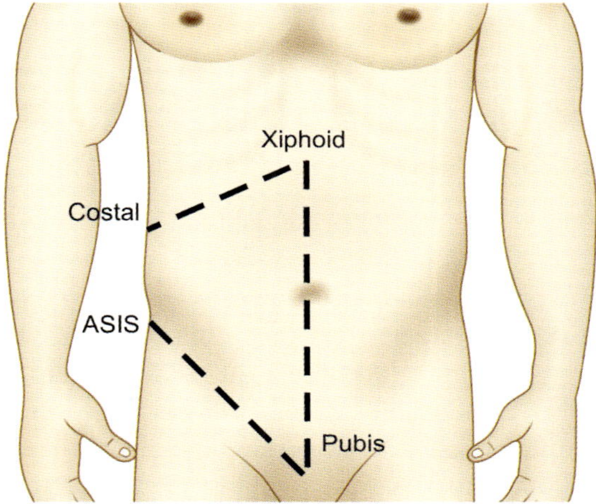

Fig. 4.8: To calculate abdominal wall surface area.

line is drawn from the anterior superior iliac spine until the costal margin is reached at the midaxillary line. The rectangle formed by the xiphopubic–pubospinal-spinocostal-costoxiphoid lines (Fig. 4.8) is measured and its area is calculated as length × breadth, and this multiplied by 2 gives an approximate surface area of the anterior abdominal wall.

$$\frac{\text{Defect surface area}}{\text{Abdominal wall surface area}} = \text{>15\% (It means always mesh repair)}$$

In patients with very pendulous abdominal walls, the surface area will be little more, e.g. in a pendulous abdomen if the circumference is 54 inches at the highest at the maximal point, then the diameter is circumference/3 which is equal to about 18 inches and the radius is 9 inches; for such a patient the surface area of the anterior abdominal wall is calculated by the formula $2\pi rh$ (h is the xiphopubic height) which gives us the complete circumferential area of the anterior and posterior abdominal walls and πrh will give us the circumference of the anterior portion alone. Then, the surface area of the defect [defect surface area (DSA)] is calculated by the product of the length and the breadth of tangential lines drawn across the surface as described previously. If the anterior abdominal wall surface area (AAWSA) divided by the DSA is more than 20% or the DSA divided AAWSA is more than 0.2 (20%) then the patient is not a good candidate for direct anatomical repair with approximation of the rectus sheath. In such patients (with large DSAs) the ensuing tension in the anterior abdominal wall will be so high that the recurrence is almost certain. Such a patient is a definite candidate for laparoscopic ventral hernioplasty.

If AAWSA/DSA greater than 20%, choose mesh only (Try to avoid anatomical repair).

PATIENTS UNDERGOING OTHER SURGERIES LAPAROSCOPICALLY—CAN THEY HAVE LAPAROSCOPIC VENTRAL HERNIA REPAIR?

The conventional teaching is that if a gallbladder or appendix or uterus is being removed in the same sitting, it is wise to avoid the possible infective complications of putting in a mesh. However, in the last 5 years (2008–2013) there has been a slew of papers justifying meshes in paracolostomy, paraileostomy, hernia repairs and indeed even in recommending that meshes be onlayed whenever an ileostomy or colostomy is closed. In the light of such a universal acceptance of mesh in contaminated situation, and in the light of the improved porosity of the newer meshes which certainly seem to have less incidences of infections, there is a global rethinking of avoiding meshes, and the authors (JSR and NS) have published papers justifying the same.

Chapter 5

The Physics of Laparoscopic Ventral Hernia Repair

THE PHYSICS BASIS OF THE VENTRAL HERNIA MESH PLASTY

In conventional open hernia repair the rectus sheath is sutured together using nonabsorbable suture material (Fig. 5.2). Every time whenever there is elevation of intra-abdominal pressure (IAP), e.g. due to coughing/sneezing, etc. the edges of the repaired defect are forced apart as the layers of the anterior abdominal wall namely posterior rectus sheath, rectus muscle, anterior rectus sheath act against the sutures (Fig. 5.1). Thus, the IAP act against the repair and this probably accounts for the high recurrence of sutured ventral hernia repair (14% in several series).

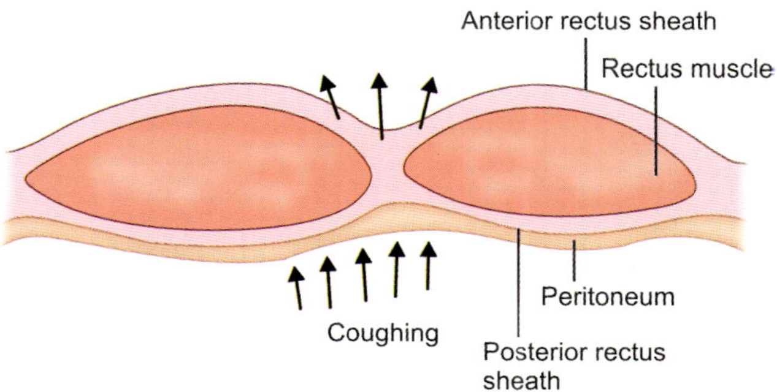

Fig. 5.1: Effect of coughing on anterior abdominal wall.

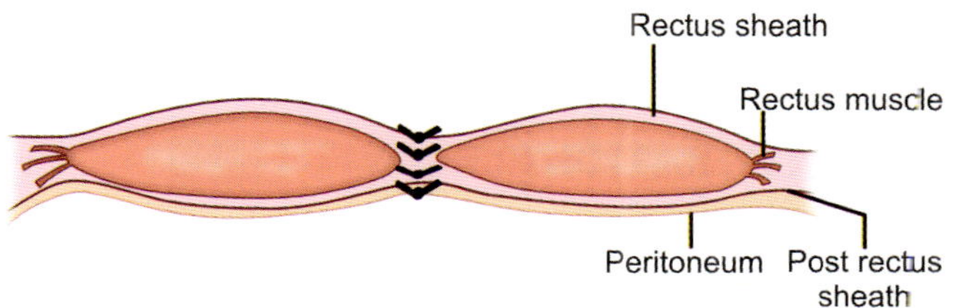

Fig. 5.2: Simple anatomical repair.

Let's see what happens in an onlay ventral hernia defect repair by mesh. If an onlay mesh of unabsorbable material like polypropylene polyester or polyamide is applied then the fibrosis induced by the fabric will heal the anterior abdominal wall and the mesh act as the buttress over the muscles. But if the patient coughs or sneezes, the IAP is increased and the layers of the anterior abdominal repairs wall act against the mesh placed over it. In both the above mentioned, the abdominal wall act against the suture line (or) onlay mesh (Fig. 5.3).

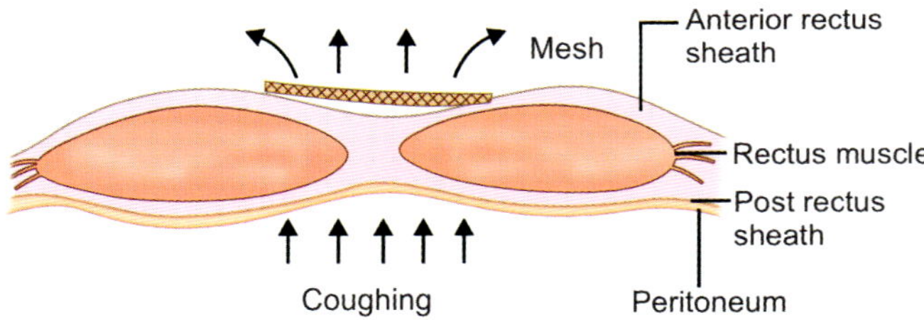

Fig. 5.3: Onlay mesh plasty and effect of coughing.

Whereas in the third situation, of lap mesh placements, mesh is anchored posterior to the peritoneum and any increase in IAP pushes the mesh. But the layers of the abdominal wall protect the transmission of the IAP against the onlay mesh. In fact the physiological usages of abdominal layers is best utilized only in a laparoscopic mesh plasty (Fig. 5.4).

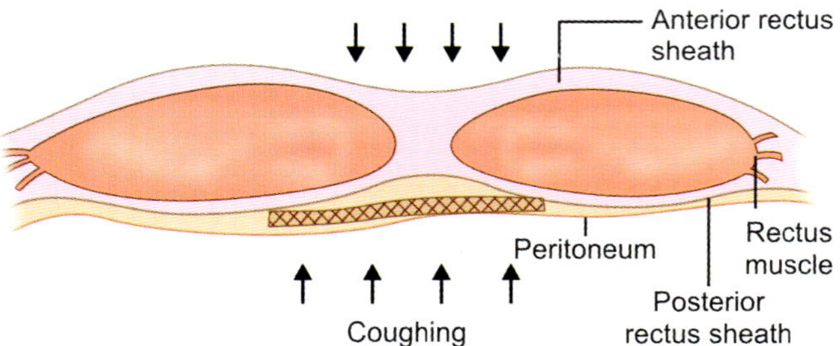

Fig. 5.4: Preperitoneal mesh placement and effect of coughing.

LAPAROSCOPIC VENTRAL HERNIA MESH PLASTY RATIONALE

Ever since the early days of laparoscopic surgery, reinforcement of the anterior abdominal wall with a prosthetic mesh applied laparoscopically, has been an attractive proposition. The earlier repairs consisted of insertion of regular polypropylene mesh (used for open ventral hernia surgeries) and fixing it with the staplers (like the PMS hernia stapler of Ethicon).

Sadly, neither the exposed polypropylene meshes nor the staplers used earlier are now deployed in the mesh repair of ventral hernias, based on the knowledge that plain polypropylene mesh exposed to small bowel causes adhesion, fistulation and enterocutaneous fistula. This has now limited the use of such meshes in such meshes in the intraperitoneal position.

The first generation of hernia staplers, such as the PMS stapler, have now been given up because of the high incidence of minor nerve entrapment between the arms of the stapler, giving rise to persistent and crippling pain around the site of the hernia mesh placement.

Chapter

6

Incisional Hernia

INTRODUCTION

The mesh fixation is identical for incisional hernia and paraumbilical hernia. However, there are some specific issues with incisional hernia that need to be addressed.

The major problem with incisional hernia surgery is the adhesiolysis before the actual hernia repair. Complex adhesions involving small bowel, large bowel and omentum can happen with multiple cheese defects, Swiss cheese defects, etc. making this one of the most difficult operations sometimes.

TECHNIQUE

Ports

The port placement for incisional hernia is based on Semm's principle, i.e. the optical port is placed as far away as possible from the edges of the defect. This can be subxiphoid or it could be in the left or right flanks (Fig. 6.1).

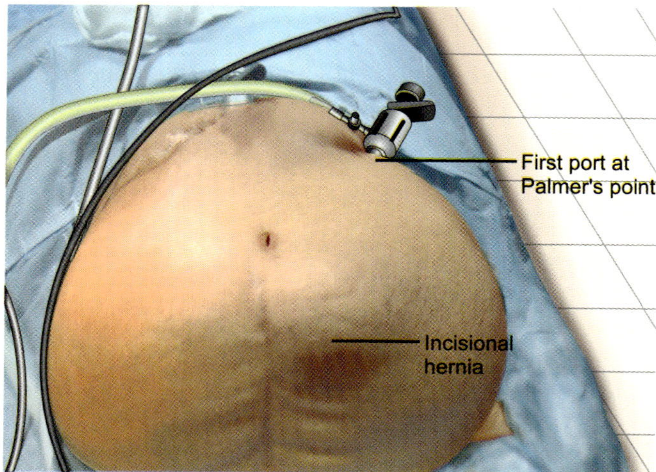

Fig. 6.1: First port placement.

A common mistake that is made is placing the port very close to the hernia defect which will not give proper visualization of the dimensions of the entire hernia gap. If the hernia has more orientation to either the left or the right side, the contralateral sides can be used for optical port entry point (Fig. 6.2).

The 30° telescope is always used after the optical port entry, and the angle of the telescope should be facing upward so as to visualize the hernia defect and the surrounding normal anterior abdominal wall.

Not only the defect but also the omentum, small bowel or large bowel contents of the sac and the adhesions also around the hernia are inspected in detail.

The adhesions are carefully lysed using all the principles of dissection described in previous chapter. Omentum and small bowel adhesions can be released using cold steel laparoscopic scissors. In case of combined omental and small bowel adhesions, the omental adhesions should be released first with the mixture of cautery or scissor dissection. Then the bowel adhesions are addressed (Figs. 6.3A and B).

In case of thick adhesions between bowels with parietal peritoneum, it should be released with cold steel laparoscopic scissor dissection along the peritoneum and posterior rectus sheath and carefully and gently dragged down toward the peritoneal cavity (Strasberg's technique).

The frequent changes of the telescope along various cannulas help to visualize the content of the sac into the hernia defect which prevent inadvertent enterotomy.

If a bowel enterotomy occurs, the best way is to close it laparoscopically and complete the adhesiolysis (*Note*: Abort the mesh part of the procedure and keep it for a subsequent date).

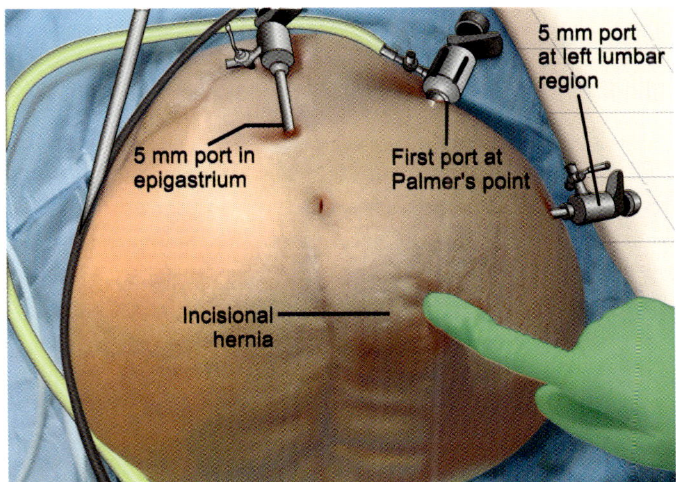

Fig. 6.2: Incisional hernia.

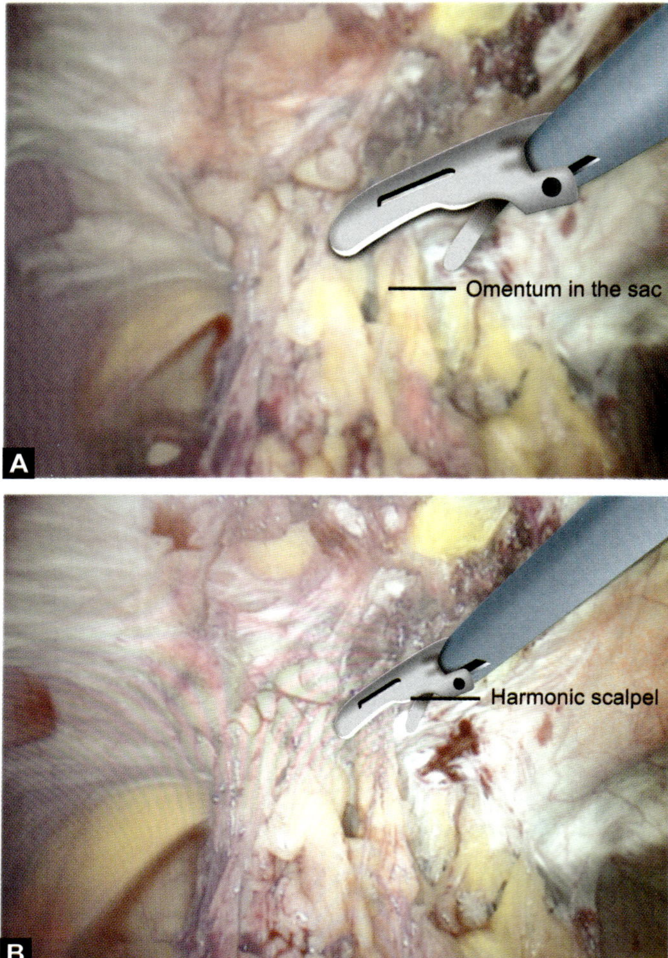

Figs. 6.3A and B: Adhesion released by harmonic scalpel.

Very often the incisional hernia defect is an asymmetrical one, which is very difficult to cover with the mesh. The technique used to cover the defect is to mark it with a spinal needle inserted at the edge of the hernia all around and to ink the skin perforations with a marker pen (Figs. 6.4A and B).

Using the glove pack paper on the defect, one can calculate the exact size of the mesh used to cover the entire hernial defect.

In case of a large hernia defect, we always recommend keeping the defect open to do tension free hernioplasty, especially if the defect edges are more than 5 cm apart in an insufflated abdominal cavity.

If an incisional hernia is situated in the lower region of the anterior abdominal wall, we sometimes access it in a transabdominal preperitoneal

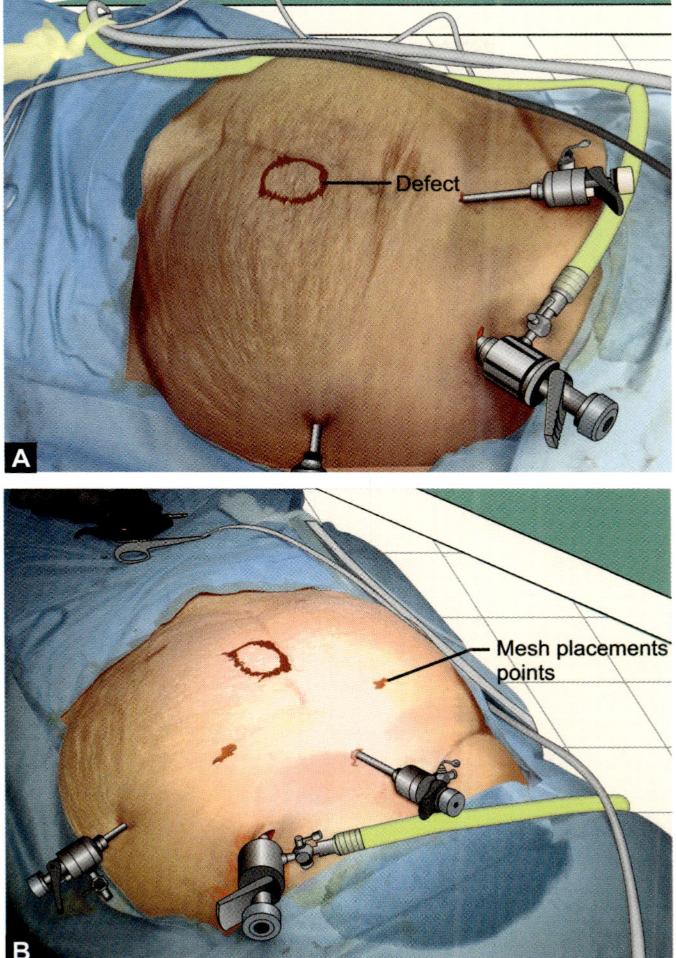

Figs. 6.4A and B: (A) Defect is marked; (B) points of mesh placement are marked.

(TAPP) pattern, widely bringing down the peritoneum, exposing the defect, taking down the sac inside the defect, putting in a regular polypropylene mesh and then closing the peritoneum once more. The major advantage of this technique is that it is extremely cost-effective.

Cost-Effective Analysis

The mesh can be tacked to the anterior abdominal wall or sutured with 1/0 polydioxanone. We prefer the latter as it is not only a far more effective way of mesh fixation, it is also very economical. On an average, about 20 sutures are required for most incisional hernias.

In addition, if the TAPP pattern is used, a regular polypropylene mesh could be deployed in place of the more expensive component separation meshes. The cost difference becomes expansive.

Tacker + Tissue component separation mesh costs around $ 860 ($ 313 + $ 547)

Suture + Tissue component separation mesh costs around $ 557 ($ 9 + $ 547).

Suture + Regular polypropylene mesh (lower abdominal incisional hernias) costs around $ 88 ($ 9 + $ 78).

Thus, in a country like India, one has to be constantly aware of cost implications of every procedure.

The titanium-coated mesh is a polypropylene mesh with an extensive coat of titanium oxide which is negatively charged to repel the small bowel adhesions. It comes at a very low cost of only $ 94–$ 109. We prefer the combination of tissue separation mesh with sutured ventral hernioplasty. This has been the most cost-effective way of fixing a ventral hernia in India today.

TAKING THE MESH INSIDE FOR APPLICATION

Here one of several techniques may be deployed:

The 9 Suture Technique (Transfascial)

In this, 9 sutures are taken on the rough (sheath) side of the mesh and are all brought out through the fascia and tied on to the sheath using the Cobbler's needle. Nine sutures are deployed, one at each corner, one centrally and one in the middle of each side of the square or rectangle as chosen. This gives a total of 9 sutures and gives a very secure fixation (Fig. 6.5).

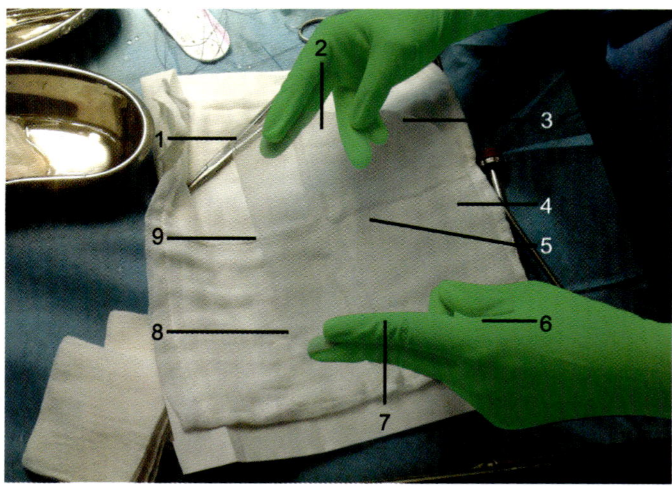

Fig. 6.5: Tissue separation mesh with 9 suture technique.

The problems with this technique are:

- It is a little more difficult than the tacker technique.
- Inadvertent involvement of one of the small nerves running in the anterior abdominal wall could cause pain in relation to the mesh.

The tacker technique is most commonly used where a double crown of tackers is deployed on the mesh, 6–8 tackers are applied in the internal crown surrounding the central areas and 12 tackers are used in the peripheries, thus giving the total of 20 tackers.

Advantage of the Tacker Technique

- It is simple and easy for beginners.

Disadvantages of Tacker Technique

- Not sure about the depth of penetration of the tackers into the anterior abdominal wall.
- Gaps in the tackers may occur permitting loops of small bowel to go inside.
- The most expensive way of fixing the mesh.

Intraperitoneal Suture Technique

This is the suture technique of our choice wherein we use 3–5 transfascial sutures to fix the edges of the mesh and put all the other sutures intraperitoneally—four sutures in the upper border and one suture in the middle of the lower edge of the mesh are all fixed transfascially and once the mesh has been fixed in place, the other sutures are all applied by intraperitoneal suturing (Fig. 6.6).

Advantage

- Inexpensive
- Gives secure fixation
- Very low risk of nerve entrapment as there is in transfascial suturing.

Disadvantage

Technically most challenging as one has to suture directly above the operative field, that is looking upward.

The mesh is taken out and rolled with the rough side in and the smooth side out, namely the intraperitoneal part of the mesh which should be outside, and the rectus sheath facing side of the mesh with all its contents in. The sutures should be within when it is put into the peritoneal cavity (Figs. 6.7 to 6.9).

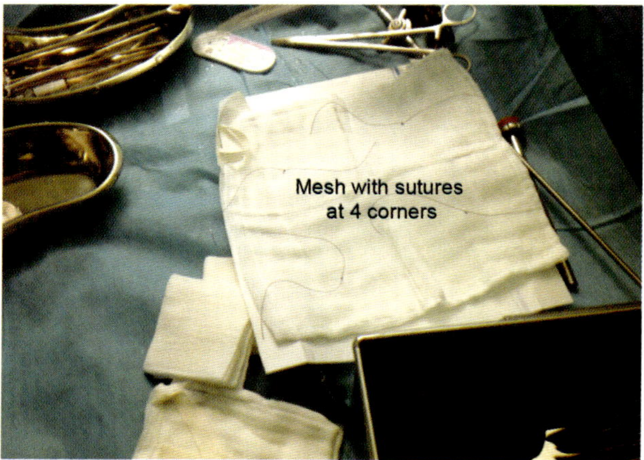

Fig. 6.6: Sutures taken at 4 corners.

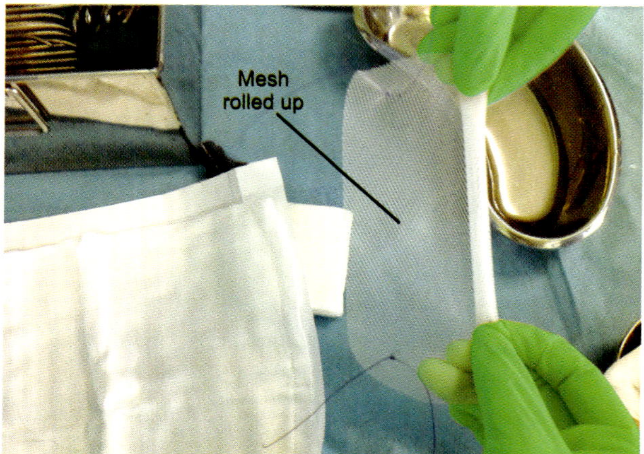

Fig. 6.7: Rolling of mesh.

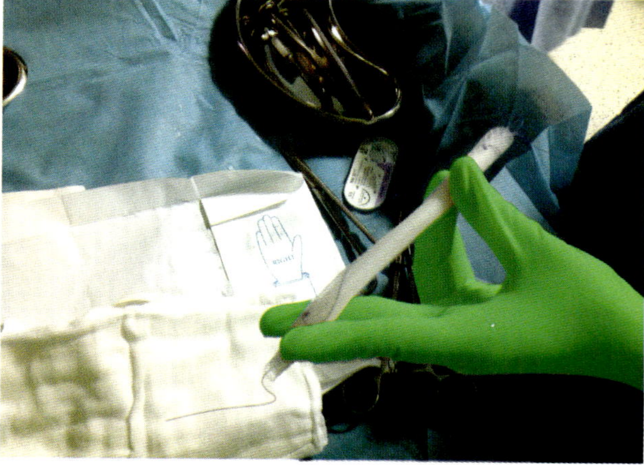

Fig. 6.8: Rolled mesh for insertion.

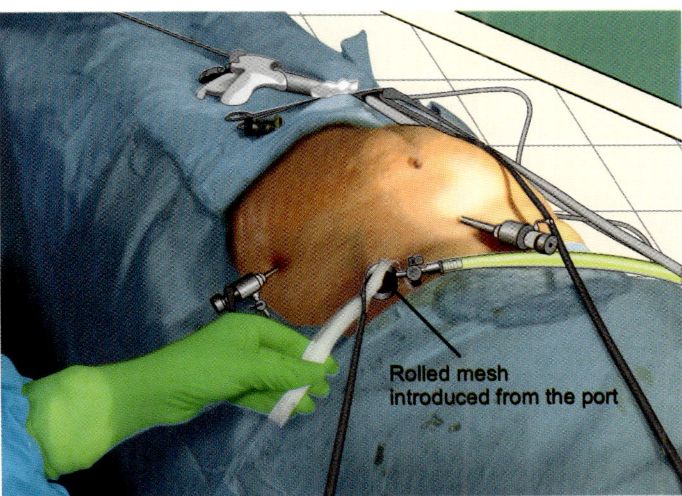

Fig. 6.9: Insertion of mesh through port.

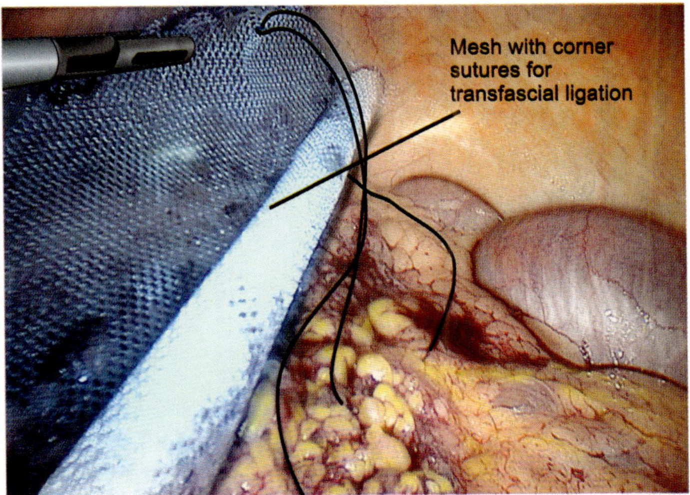

Fig. 6.10: Mesh introduction and rolled mesh inside abdomen.

When transfascial suturing is done the two tails of the suture should be 7 cm in length. This is the ideal length for picking it up and taking it up even in obese patients (Fig. 6.10).

The mesh is introduced holding the grasper through the 12 mm port into the peritoneal cavity.

The mesh is unrolled inside the peritoneal cavity with the rough side facing the anterior abdominal wall and the smooth side facing the omentum and small bowel.

The following technique is used to lift up the tails beyond the anterior abdominal wall:

- A 2 mm nick is made with 11 blade at the proposed site of the mesh fixation.
- Cobbler's needle is put into that and opened up intra abdominally. This is done by the second assistant or scrub nurse.

The "Garland" Technique

- Using a grasper in each hand, the tail is grasped, with one hand holding the tip of the tail and one hand holding the body of the tail 2–3 cm from the tip. The left and right hand together garland the open limbs of the tips of the Cobbler's needle. The Cobbler's needle closes, grasping the tail, and the thread is brought out and held on with an artery forceps (Figs. 6.11A to C). Now the Cobbler's needle is passed again through same cutaneous opening but into the sheath 3 mm–4 mm from the primary entry point and the process is repeated with the next tail (Figs. 6.11D and E).
- The two tails are tied down on the sheath leaving a little bit of air between the knot and the anterior abdominal wall (air knotting) (Fig. 6.11F).
- This process is repeated at 9 points all around including the center to fix the mesh in the transfascial technique.

Partially Sutured Technique

Three sutures are tied transfascially on the upper edge of the mesh and one suture is tied in the central aspect of the lower border of the mesh. Then a 1/0 or 2/0 polyamide (nylon) or polypropylene (prolene) or polydioxanone is taken in through the 12 mm cannula.

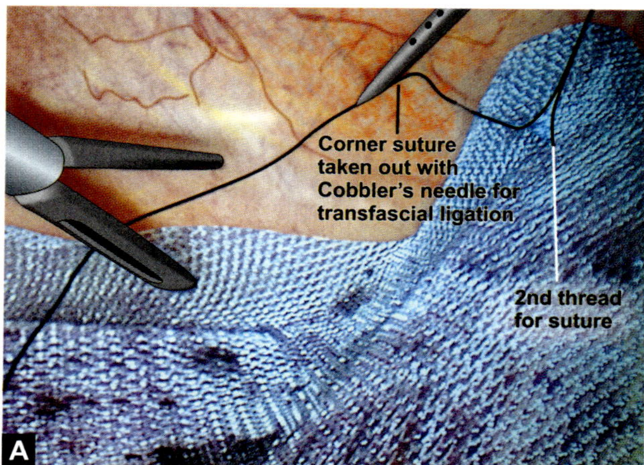

Fig. 6.11A

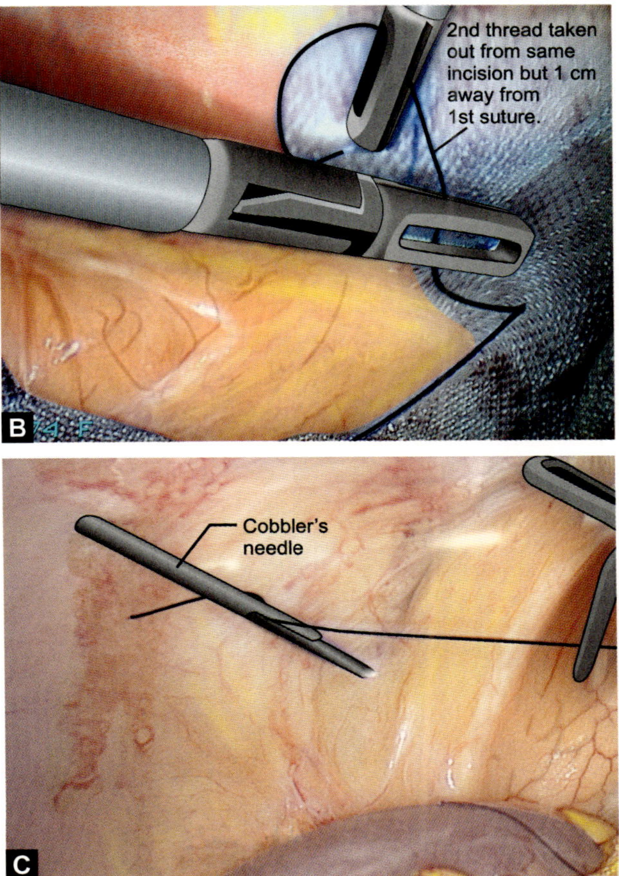

Figs. 6.11A to C: Transfascial ligation of corners of mesh with Cobbler's needle.

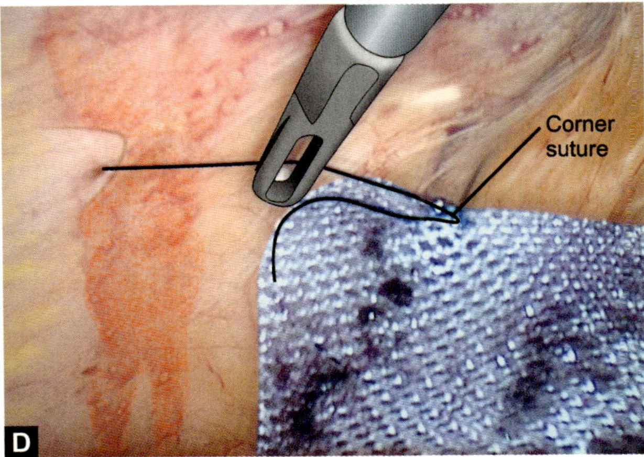

Fig. 6.11D

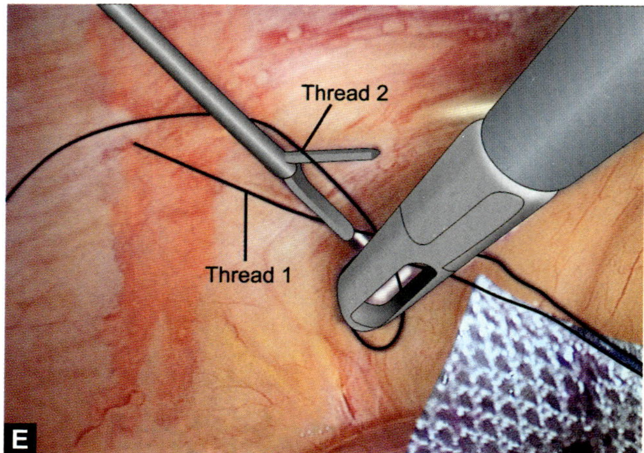

Figs. 6.11D and E: Transfascial ligation through 2 separate points.

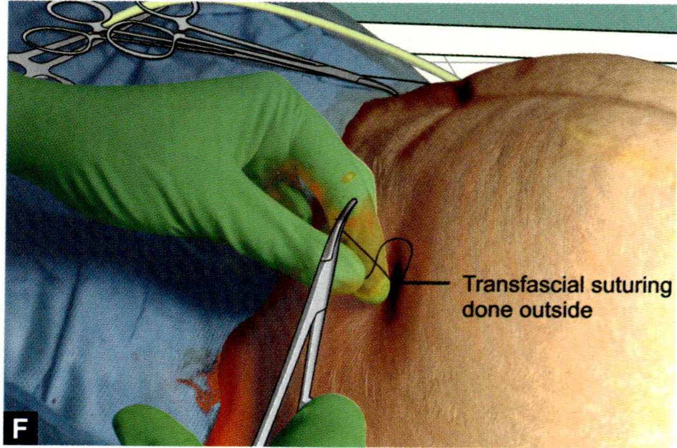

Fig. 6.11F: Air knotting.

Interrupted sutures are applied at 2 cm intervals starting from the two lower corners of the mesh coming up all the way along the sides until the entire mesh is fixed to the inner aspect of the anterior abdominal wall.

Tacker Technique

In the tacker technique, the mesh is taken in without any suture and a tacker is applied to the center of the mesh and to a point just above the center of the defect. To prevent the tacker from going subcutaneous counter pressure is applied with a palm externally on the anterior abdominal wall and the tacker is fired. Then the tacker is fired at the four corners of the mesh, about 1 cm from the border (Fig. 6.12A).

At this point, one must stress that all corner and side sutures should be taken about 1 cm away from the edge of the mesh. This prevent recurrence of the hernia in case shrinkage of the mesh happens at that point (Figs. 6.12B to D).

As the lower border is being sutured either transfascially or by direct suturing, the intraperitoneal gas pressure is brought down from 12 mm to 7 mm or 8 mm to ensure smooth fixation of the mesh to the inner aspect of the anterior abdominal wall (Fig. 6.12E).

It is much more ergonomically difficult if one has to suture the upper edge of the mesh and this is why we like to finish the upper edge with the full pneumoperitoneum before moving down to the lower edge of the mesh.

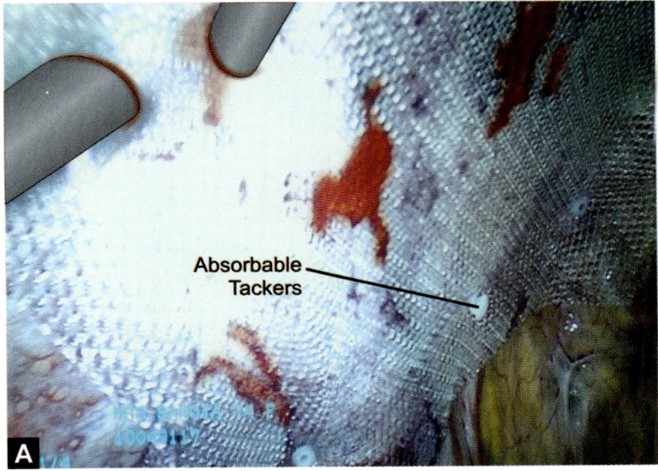

Fig. 6.12A: Fixing the mesh with absorbable tackers.

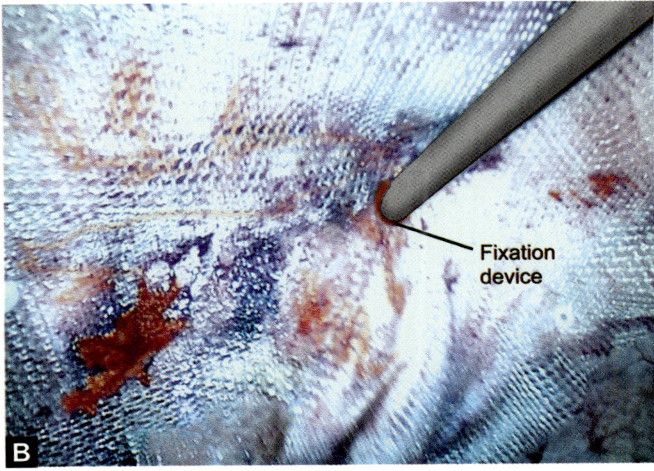

Fig. 6.12B

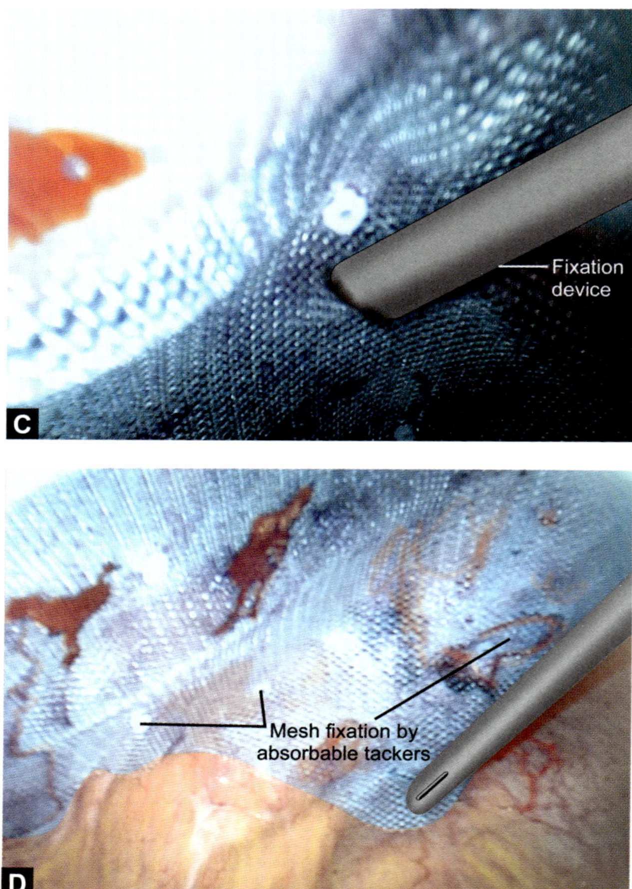

Figs. 6.12B to D: Mesh fixation by tackers.

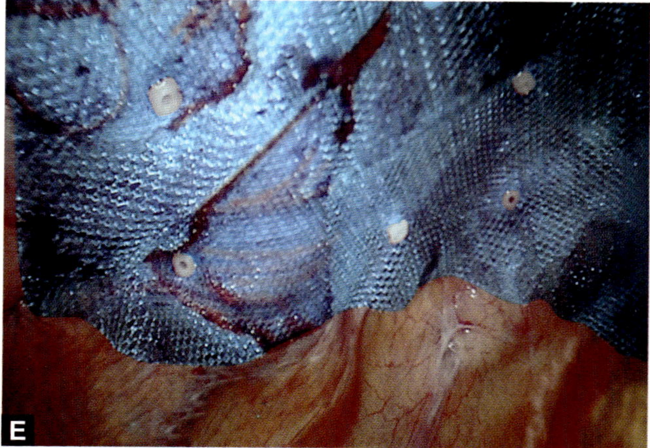

Fig. 6.12E: Double crown technique.

The upper edge being very close to the telescope and camera always be more difficult ergonomically to work on.

Technique of Ventral Hernia

First, we deal with paraumbilical hernias, epigastric hernias and divarication of the recti. The reason is that the technique is identical for these three conditions.

Position

Patient is kept in the supine position with the arms tucked by the side. A slight head end elevation of 30° is given to allow the small bowel to gravitate toward the pelvis. The surgeon stands above right shoulder of the patient (Fig. 6.13).

Trocars and Ports

The first port or the optic port is introduced in the subxiphoid area, about 1–2 inches below the tip of the xiphoid process. This is usually a 12 mm port allowing optics and also allowing the passage of the needle and thread and also the rolled up mesh. The left hand working port and right hand working port are both in identical position 1 inch in front of the anterior axillary line and 1 inch below the costal margin. It is important that the left and right hand working ports are far away from the right and left mid clavicular lines so that there should be no ergonomic difficulty in suturing the mesh. The first assistant (camera person) stands to the left of the patient's head (behind the left shoulder) (Fig. 6.14).

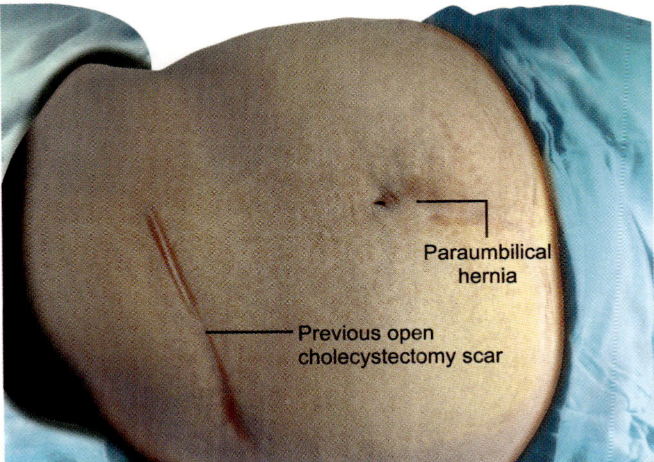

Fig. 6.13: Position of patient.

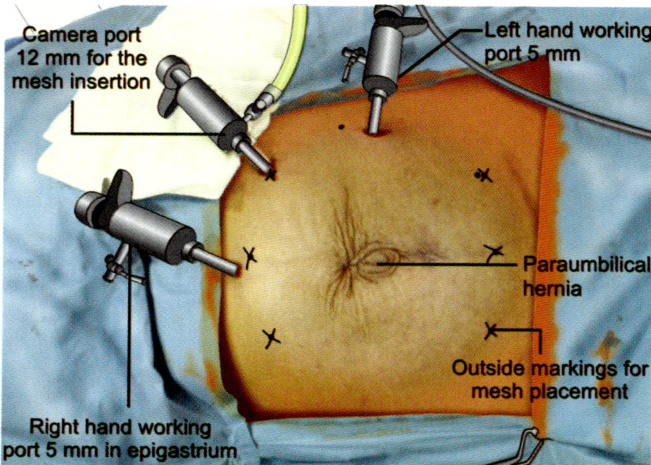

Fig. 6.14: Ports paraumbilical hernia.

Initially after the pneumoperitoneum is created, the edges of the fascial defect are examined and if any omentum is passing in this, is reduced. The left hand working port carries a nontoothed grasper (bowel grasper) and the right hand does the adhesiolysis if required with the scissors and cautery.

After the omentum (or any other content) is taken down, the sac inside the hernia is dealt with. The reason for this is that, leaving the sac might result in an uncomfortable seroma, with the patient wondering if the hernia was done at all! There are two ways of dealing with the sac inside the defect.

It can be thermoobliterated by burning it with the hook or spatula or Maryland's forceps. The sac can be pulled back and completely excised from the subcutaneous fat and sheath.

After the sac has been dealt with, the edges of the mesh are marked out. This is done by going 5 cm outside the visible edge of the defect above and below and the edges are marked with diathermy (this is called scoring the peritoneum). This is done before the sheath edge is closed, as the mesh should occupy 5 cm beyond the fascial defect "before closure".

When the fascial defect is closed, this procedure limits seroma formation but otherwise adds no significant strength to the placement of mesh.

Approximately 1–2 mm incision is made below the fascial defect and 1-0 nylon suture or a polypropylene suture is passed through this regular needle holder and the needle passed into the peritoneal cavity, this is seen visualized laparoscopically and pull through then a series of continuous sutures are applied to the sheath edge on both sides from below upward until the upper edge of the fascial defect is reached.

When this is reached the suture is pulled tight and then another series of sutures are applied to the edges coming from above down below until the lower edge of the fascial defect is reached, then a Cobbler's needle is passed through the same skin incision but to enter the peritoneal cavity about 3–5 mm from the original entry point of the needle and the thread and needle have grasped between the limbs of the Cobbler's needle and brought outside the abdomen.

When both tails are grasped and traction applied the fascial edges come together giving a flat appearance of anterior abdominal wall. Then the sutures applied to the anterior abdominal wall sheath which serves to completely close the defect. We recommend fascial closure in defects less than 3 cm wide as the tension of the anterior abdominal wall increases if larger defects are suture closed.

Two pictures one is starting to close the defect and second is after the closure of defect.

Choice of Mesh in Ventral Hernia Repair

There are many types of meshes and there is a bewildering array for the surgeon to choose from, but the major principles will be dealt here and the most common meshes in use will be described in detail.

The principle of the meshes is to allow incorporation of fibroblastic proliferation and a dense collagenous matrix which strengthen the anterior abdominal wall. But unlike an onlay mesh where any nonabsorbable material like polypropolene or polyamide would serve as a lattice work to have the extracellular matrix led down by the fibroblast, in ventral hernia meshplasty it is important to prevent the major complication of bowel adhering to the mesh. Several case series have been consistently documented when the regular polypropolene or polyester meshes are exposed to small bowel dangerous adhesions and fistulation and multiple abscesses could result.

In order to offset this dangerous complication, research produced a number of meshes that were acceptable for the intraperitoneal onlay mesh (IPOM) technique.

Principle

The main principle of all these meshes is the intensely negatively charged serosa of the small bowel, as the serosa of the bowel is very rich in electrons. Most of the meshes are positively charged and this causes an immediate attraction of the small bowel surface to the foreign body. This can be offset by adding another layer to the mesh that is strongly negative charged, which consequently repel the small bowel, and prevent mesh adhesions to small bowel.

Chapter 7

Meshes and Fixation Devices in Laparoscopic Ventral Hernia Repairs

SOME PROPERTIES OF MESHES

Macroporosity

Large pores in the mesh permit the ingrowth of fibroblasts, contributing to a healthy perimesh scar. This is very desirable.

Incidentally, the less of unabsorbable textile equals less gram weight of the mesh, with lesser postsurgical pain. High porosity meshes are Ultrapro (Ethicon) and Parietex™ (Covidien).

Microporosity

The weave of the mesh allows interstices in most meshes, but not in textiles like Gor-Tex® or Teflon® [polytetrafluoroethylene (PTFE)].

If the interstices contain gaps of more than 10 microns, even if the mesh gets infected, it can be washed and cleaned, and white blood cells (WBCs), with a diameter of 7–9 microns can reach the bacteria (with a diameter of 1 micron).

On the other hand, with PTFE, with a 1–2 micron gap, the bacteria will permanently lodge as WBCs cannot reach them. Therefore, such meshes need to be removed.

Mesh Shrinkage

It is now known that polypropylene meshes can shrink by nearly 30% of their size, accounting for recurrence. This factor should be taken into account when covering the defect, ensuring an overlap of 3–5 cm.

Also, tacking or suturing to the edges of the mesh should be done at least 1 cm away from the edge to avoid loss of fixation with shrinkage.

Technically, the process is fibrosis plus mesh with contraction and is actually called "mesh-scar contraction".

Molecular Weight of Meshes

"Dalton" is the term used to denote grams per mole of tissue. If the weight of a mesh is less than 40 Dalton, it is known as low molecular weight mesh. If the weight of a mesh is 40–80 Dalton, it is called moderate weight and above 80 Dalton, high molecular weight.

Higher the weight, more the incidence of postsurgical pain or "inguinodynia". The cognizance of this fact has spawned a new generation low-molecular-weight meshes, always preferable in inguinal hernias.

TYPES OF MESHES

Parietex™ Composite Mesh (Covidien)

This entire set of meshes is called tissue separation meshes as they serve to separate the intraperitoneal tissues from the anterior abdominal wall. The meshes and principles are as follows: the Parietex™ composite mesh (Covidien, TN) involves polyester on the side facing the anterior abdominal wall and involves polyethylene glycol and collagen hydrogel on the inner aspect; the collagen hydrogel is negatively charged and repels the small bowel (Fig. 7.1).

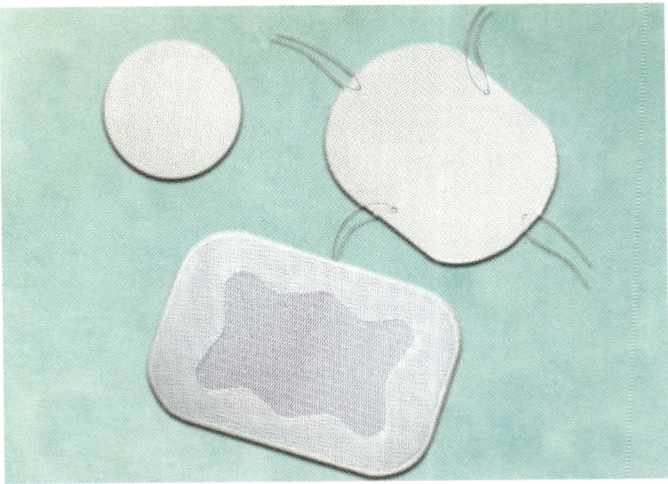

Fig. 7.1: Parietex™ composite mesh (Covidien, TN).

Sepramesh™ (Bard)

The Sepramesh™ (Bard) consists of polypropylene on top and facing the rectus sheath and polyethylene glycol and glycerol on the inner aspect facing the small bowel (Fig. 7.2).

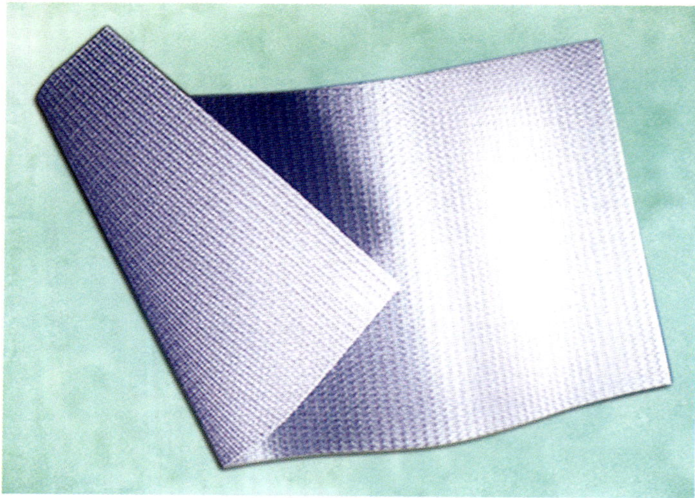

Fig. 7.2: Sepramesh™ (Bard).

Proceed® Mesh (Ethicon)

Proceed® Mesh (Ethicon) is a four-layered mesh. The upper layer is one of polydioxanone suture (PDS), the second layer contains polypropylene, the third layer is once more PDS and the fourth layer is the intraperitoneal layer containing oxidized regenerated cellulose (ORC) (Fig. 7.3).

There is the Pro-Visc (Lotus) which contains polypropylene on the upper surface and polyvinyl chloride (PVC) on the lower surface; there is

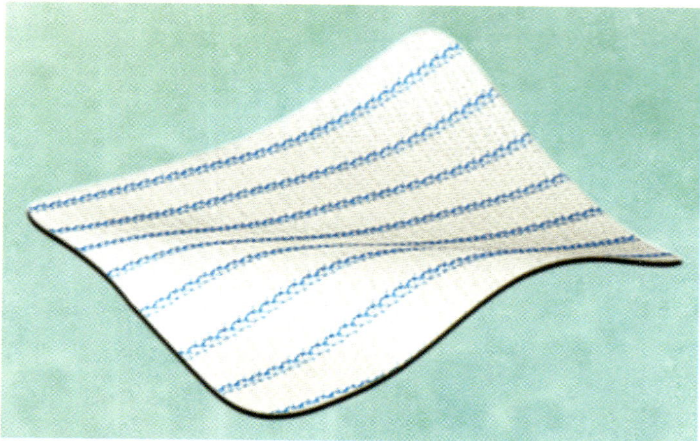

Fig. 7.3: The Proceed® Mesh.

the popular dual mesh which contains polypropylene facing the posterior rectus sheath and an expanded PTFE to face the small bowel.

There is also the less frequently available meshes include the L mesh which contains expanded PTFE facing the small bowel and low-density polyethylene which is very porous facing the posterior rectus sheath.

All these meshes include the anti-adhesion barrier facing the peritoneal surface, the latest mesh is called the FlexHD® mesh which actually uses a cellular human dermis on the inner aspect and polypropylene on the superior aspect. The biological meshes like the FlexHD® and the BIOSIS are only mentioned here for completion as they are not usually deployed in a ventral hernia. The biological meshes usually contain porcine, small intestinal submucosa or bovine pericardium and the idea of biological meshes is that they allow extracellular matrix to fill in the interstices of the biological mesh with new vessels they lay down and orderly template for remodeling of the collagen fibers in that areas and are used in contaminated are dirty wounds, especially when infected meshes are removed and a simple suture repair is deemed insufficient.

C-QUR™ mesh (Atrium) which contains polypropylene on the upper surface and contains omega-3 fatty acids on the inner aspect which is once more strongly negatively charged (Fig. 7.4).

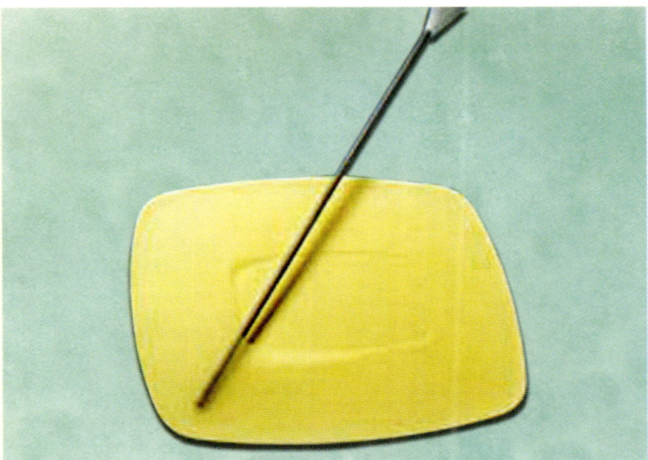

Fig. 7.4: The C-QUR™ mesh (Atrium).

Pro-Visc (Lotus): This makes use of a polyurethane (PVC) surface to coat the bowel to face the bowel and polyester surface to face the rectus sheath (Fig. 7.5).

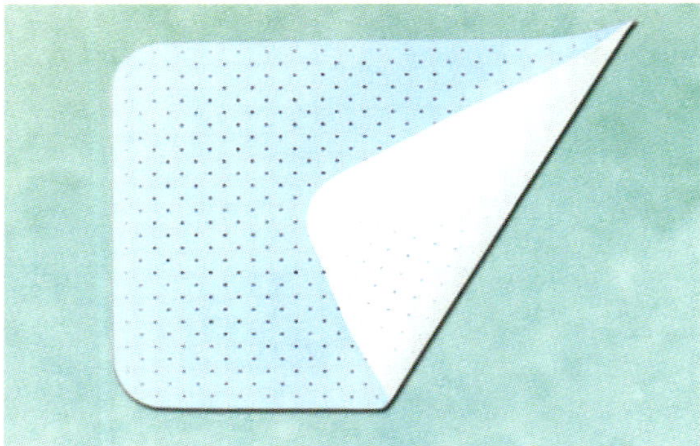

Fig. 7.5: Pro-Visc (Lotus).

Physiomesh® (Ethicon): This mesh has four layers; a polypropylene layer that has sandwiched by two layers of PDS and fourth deeper layer which is made up of ORC (Fig. 7.6).

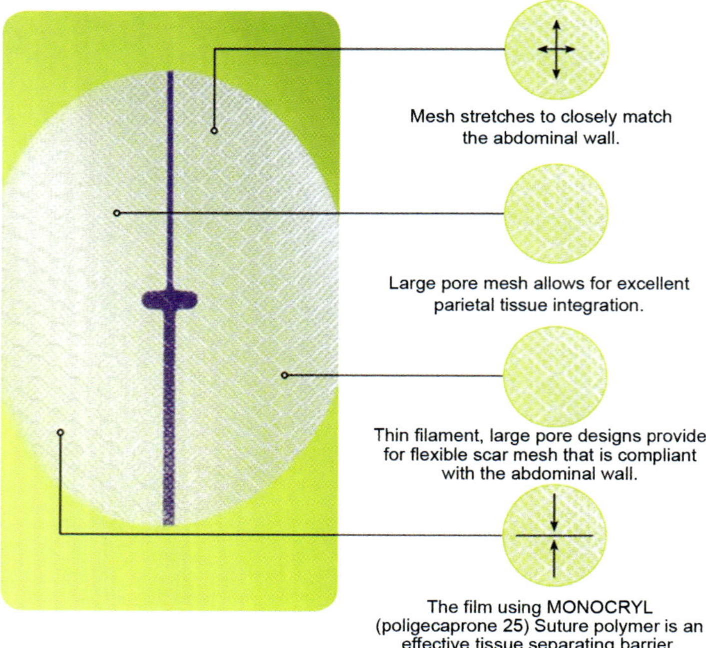

Fig. 7.6: Physiomesh® (Ethicon).

The advantage of tacker device is the simple technique for the beginner but the problems of the tackers are: in patients with very obese abdominal walls, the fixation might not be very good (*see* below for differing depths of fixation devices). The most important issue is the cost of tackers on average. Each tacker costs about $ 16 and securing a double ring of tackers, so-called double crown technique, would involve nearly 20 tackers amounting to $ 313 can be offset by employing suturing with polypropylene on nylon which would amount to the total of $ 3. Thus, there is a 100 times saving the cost! The earlier staplers have been withdrawn and there are three or four tackers available commonly; the most common in use is the ProTack from Covidien which comes in disposable units of unhandled plus cartridge of 20 (Fig. 7.7). A newer absorbable tacker by the same company, made out of PDS, is also available and has obvious advantages of not remaining permanently as foreign body.

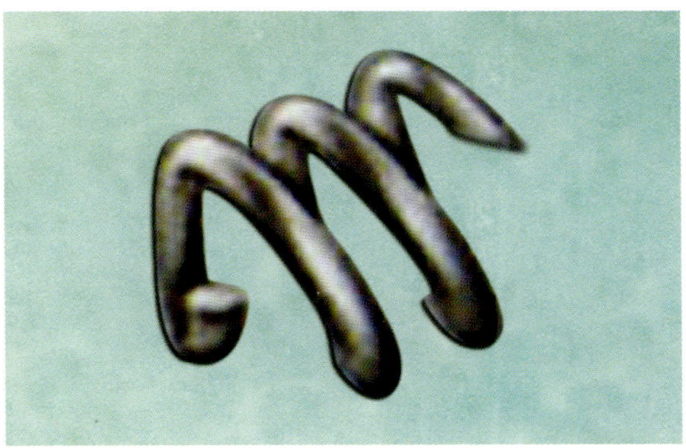

Fig. 7.7: ProTack (Covidien).

Secure Strap® (Ethicon) both absorbable and nonabsorbable tackers are available from Ethicon (Fig. 7.8).

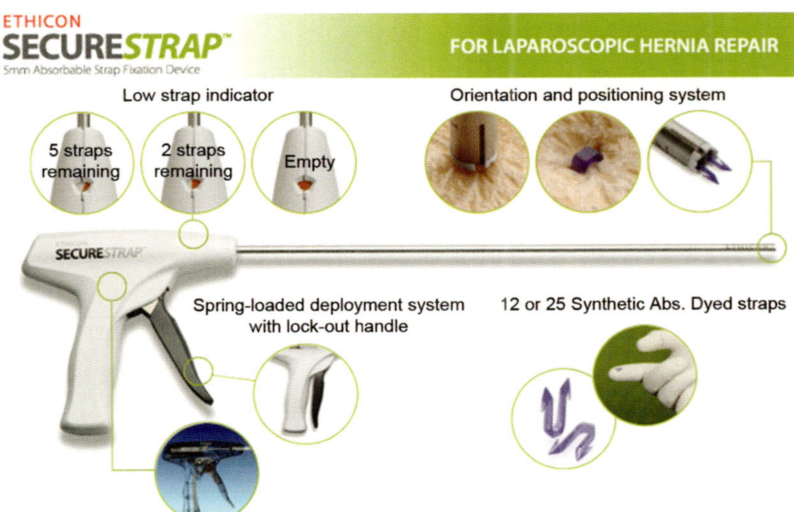

Fig. 7.8: Secure Strap® (Ethicon).

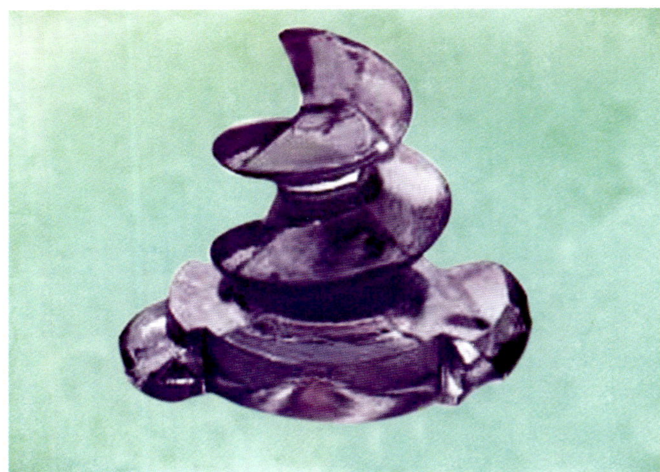

Fig. 7.9: SorbaFix™ (Bard).

Bard Syntack is the one with a deepest penetration into the anterior abdominal wall and therefore technically probably the safest tacker to be used. However, all the tackers are expensive ways of fixation of mesh and that is why we have increasingly moved away from tackers. Tackers are used in patients where the mesh needs to be fixed quickly (Fig. 7.9).

8

Spigelian Hernia

INTRODUCTION

This hernia is named after Adriaan Van Den Spiegel, who described the semilunar line as one which runs from the tip of the 9th costal cartilage vertically down up to the pubic spine and contributes to Spigelian hernia by lateral edges of rectus abdominal muscle. The hernia was first described by Klinkosch in 1764. These hernias are very rare, constituting approximately 0.1% of abdominal wall hernias.

PATHOPHYSIOLOGY

It is said that the perforating vessels of the inferior epigastric cause weakening of the fascia at the semilunar line. A small amount of preperitoneal fat enters here which gradually leads to hernia. This hernia has also been described as a complication of chronic ambulatory peritoneal dialysis (CAPD). Obesity, multiparity and multiple operations in the lower abdominal wall seems to contribute to the formation of a Spigelian hernia.

SPIGELIAN HERNIA BELT

This is an area that is 0–6 cm cranial to interspinous plane. About 90% of Spigelian hernias occur in this belt, the remaining occurring between 6 cm and 9 cm from the interspinous plane.

The danger of Spigelian hernia is that it is a well-defined defect in the aponeurosis which is sharp. The omentum of bowel passing through the hernia sac is more liable for strangulation and often lies in an interparietal plane resulting in delayed diagnosis and even on strangulation at presentation.

The Spigelian hernia occurs through a slit-like defect in the abdominal wall adjacent to the semilunar line in the lower abdomen where the posterior sheath is deficient.

REPAIR OF SPIGELIAN HERNIA

There are three techniques to repair Spigelian hernias. Depending on the situation and anatomy inside any of the repairs can be selected by the surgeon. The following are the three methods to do that.

1. Laparoscopic intraperitoneal onlay mesh (IPOM)
2. The laparoscopic transabdominal preperitoneal (TAPP) technique
3. The laparoscopic total extraperitoneal (TEP) technique.

In view of the peritoneum usually being redundant in the supravesical area where this hernia occurs, we tend to prefer the TAPP technique. In patients with multiple surgeries were the peritoneum is scarred and stretched, we prefer an IPOM technique exactly as described in the previous section on the paraumbilical hernia.

The main difference in the technique in the IPOM is that the edges of the defect in the aponeurosis can often be closed with suturing of the posterior sheath being done from lateral to medial and back again to the lateral end. But if the defect is more than 2 cm suturing is not advisable, as it will give tension to the tissues.

Following this, we lay one of the tissue separation meshes like Parietex composite, Provisk, C-QUR or the proceed, and fix either with the tacker or transfascial ligation augmented by intraperitoneal suturing as described above.

As we have already described TAPP and TEP techniques in previous chapters here we are describing the IPOM technique.

LAPAROSCOPIC INTRAPERITONEAL ONLAY MESH PLASTY

Trocars are inserted, with the optical trocar being 10–15 cm superior to the superior edge of the hernia. This is the optical port and also the port that will take the mesh and is usually 12 mm port.

The right hand working port is inserted one hands breadth lateral to the optical port and 1 inch inferior to it.

Similarly, the left hand working port inserts one hands breadth lateral to the optical port and 1 inch below the same.

This gives a good triangulation for ergonomic dissection.

The hernia contents are first reduced into the abdomen (Fig. 8.1).

This might require some "taxis" or pressure from outside, combined with traction from the intraperitoneal aspect (Fig. 8.2).

When the hernia contents are reduced, the edges of the defect are clearly made out (Fig. 8.3).

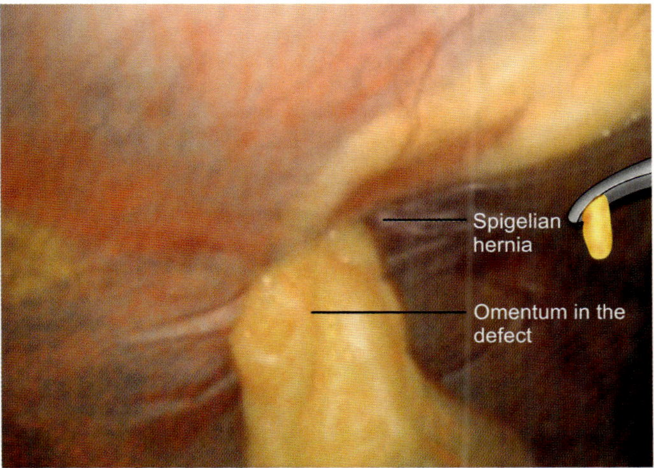

Fig. 8.1: Spigelian hernia with omentum in the defect.

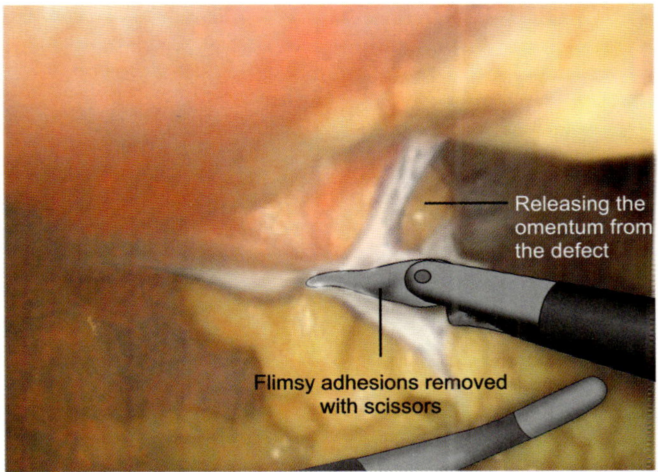

Fig. 8.2: Releasing the omentum from the defect.

After the hernia contents are reduced if the size of defect is more than 3 cm, then there is no need to suture the defect from inside. Size of defect is calculated and mesh size is selected. For 3 cm defect we need to use at least 15 × 15 size mesh.

Mesh is rolled and pushed inside from 12 mm port (Fig. 8.4).

All four corners of mesh suture are tied for transfascial ligation of mesh.

Rest of mesh is fixed by tackers (Figs. 8.5 to 8.7).

Mesh is fixed by double crown technique (Figs. 8.8 and 8.9).

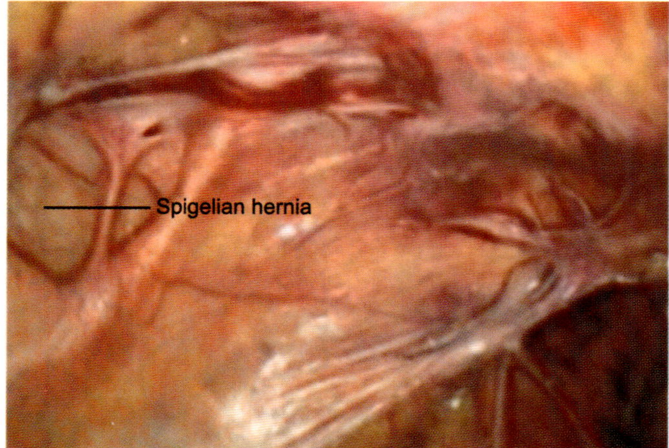

Fig. 8.3: Spigelian hernia after reduction of omental contents.

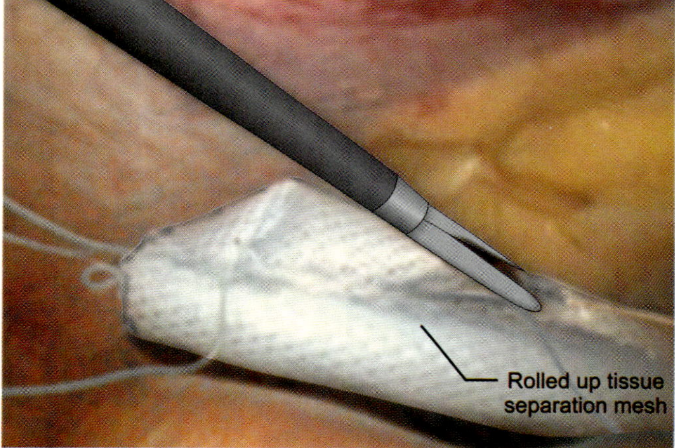

Fig. 8.4: Introduction of tissue separation mesh.

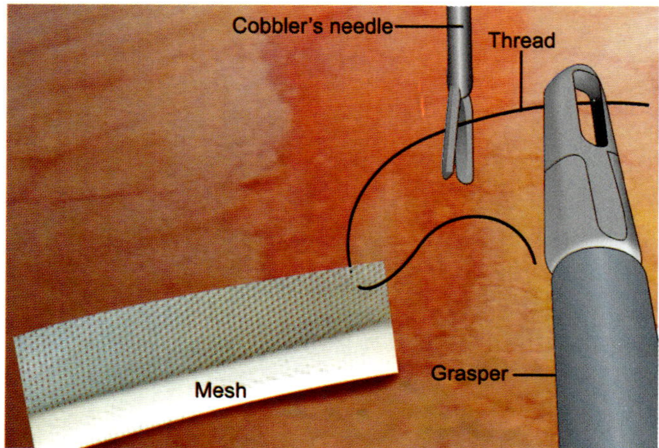

Fig. 8.5: Technique of Transfascial ligation of mesh.

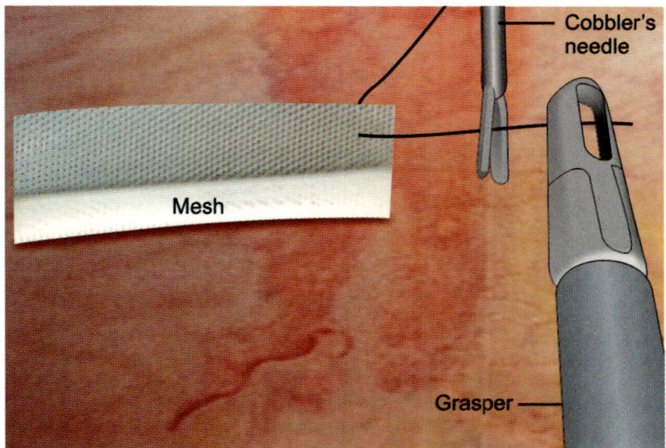

Fig. 8.6: Technique of taking 2nd suture with Cobbler's needle.

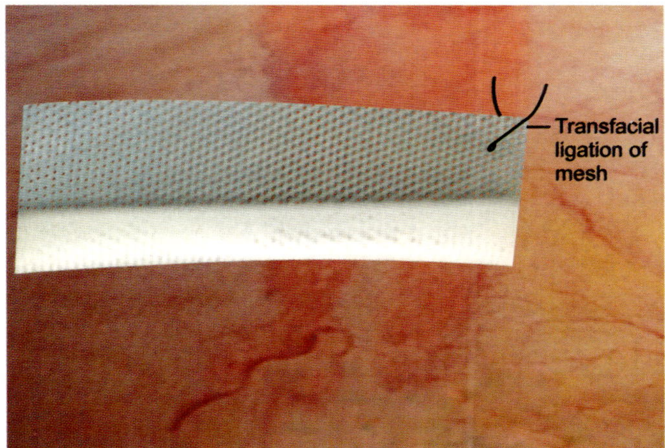

Fig. 8.7: Both sutures taken through anterior abdominal wall.

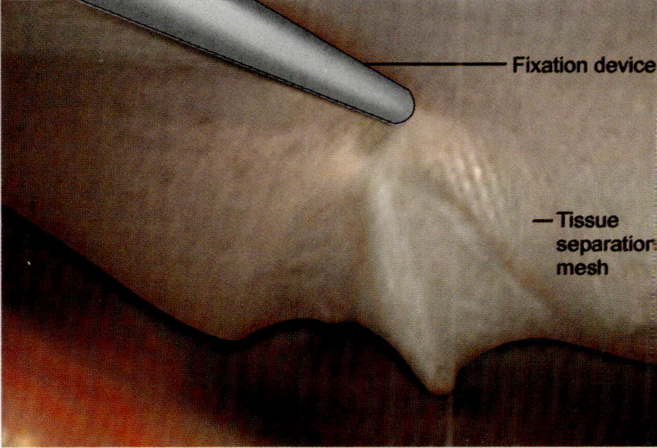

Fig. 8.8: Fixation of mesh with fixation device.

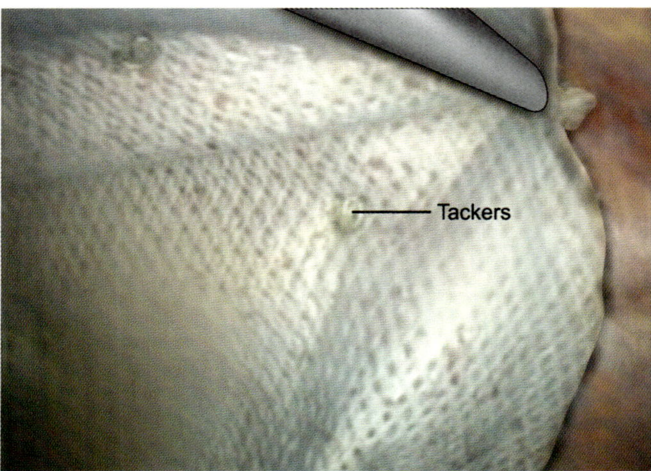

Fig. 8.9: Double crown technique.

LAPAROSCOPIC TAPP TECHNIQUE

A transverse cut is made, starting from 5 cm from lateral edge of the defect and extending up to a point 7 cm medial to the edge of the defect. Where it approaches the defect, the peritoneal incision curves downward toward the edge of the defect. Then the peritoneal flap is extensively raised above and below until the edge of the defect is completely exposed all around.

The dissection proceeds for about 7 cm superiorly and 7–10 cm inferiorly.

The inferior is extent of the dissection is taken up to the pubic ramus and extended laterally as it is done for TAPP hernia.

When the peritoneal closure is completed the entire defect is been covered with polypropylene mesh and no part of the mesh is visible to the telescope from the peritoneal cavity, thus avoiding the possible trap of adhesion.

Index

Page numbers followed by *f* refer to figure.

N

O

P

R

S

T